Praise for Terry McDermott's

101 Theory Drive

"A fascinating portrait of one brilliant, eccentric scientist and an insight into some of the groundbreaking science that seeks to explain memory." —*San Francisco Book Review*

"A fun read about some fascinating neuroscience, and, even more importantly, provides a rare look into how science is really done." —Leonard Mlodinow, author of *The Drunkard's Walk*

"This is an engrossing story of science and the brilliant, flawed people who make it." —*Publishers Weekly*

"A stirring account of how important scientific research gets done." —*Kirkus*

"Engrossing. . . . A book about the truth, and the endless human struggle to find it." —Jonah Lehrer, author of *How We Decide*

"Thrilling. . . . A story you won't forget." —David Eagleman, author of *Sum*

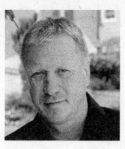

TERRY McDERMOTT

101 Theory Drive

Terry McDermott is a former national reporter for the *Los Angeles Times* and the author of *Perfect Soldiers: The 9/11 Hijackers—Who They Were, Why They Did It*. He lives in Southern California.

101 Theory Drive

The Discovery of Memory

Terry McDermott

Vintage Books
A Division of Random House, Inc.
New York

For lab rats everywhere
of however many legs

Memory is a net: one that finds it full of fish when he takes it from the brook, but a dozen miles of water have run through it without sticking.

—Oliver Wendell Holmes

Contents

101 Theory Drive

CHAPTER ONE

The Talking Cure

THE ENGRAM

Save for Lynch, Lynch Lab was empty the day I arrived, a clear blue winter morning in the last week of December 2004. Outside, the parking lot contained nothing but clean black asphalt and bright white lines. Inside, the double ranks of stainless-steel lab benches were bare and quiet. Much to Gary Lynch's chagrin, every single one of the dozen or so scientists, students, and technicians who worked in the lab had gone on holiday. Lynch's attitude toward other people's vacations could most charitably be described as dim. He worked 365 days a year. Why couldn't they? Especially now.

Scientists in Lynch's lab at the University of California, Irvine, had recently developed a technique that Lynch, a neuroscientist who had been investigating the biochemistry of memory for more than thirty years, thought would allow researchers for the first time to visualize a trace of memory; that is, to see a map of the physical changes in the brain that occur when a memory is made. This was not an insignificant undertaking. For at least a century, scientists had been trying—and failing—to do exactly what Lynch thought his lab was on the verge of accomplishing: to teach an animal a new skill or experience; to, in other words, expose that animal's brain to something in the exterior world, then look deeply enough into the close, dark, complicated space that is the mammalian brain and say, with certainty, "There! Right there! That's it." "The thing itself," Lynch sometimes called it, making it sound like a rumored but never-quite-glimpsed spirit in the night.

Such a physical trace of memory is commonly called an engram. Karl Lashley, a famed American psychologist, had popularized the term in the mid-twentieth century and had devoted a significant portion of his career to pursuing it. His search had been exhaustive and, in the end, fruitless.

"This series of experiments has yielded a good bit of information about what and where the memory trace is not," Lashley wrote. "It has discovered nothing directly of the real nature of the engram. I sometimes feel, in reviewing the evidence on the localization of the memory trace, that the necessary conclusion is that learning just is not possible. It is difficult to conceive of a mechanism that can satisfy the conditions set for it. Nevertheless, in spite of such evidence against it, learning sometimes does occur."

The history of memory research since Lashley had been rife with heated disagreements about whether such a thing as an engram actually existed, about whether such a thing could actually be seen, about what such a thing would look like if it did exist and could be seen, about where it would be, and, especially, about what did or did not occur inside the brain cells, called neurons, that would cause such a thing to exist. If, that is, it did.

Of course, Lashley's original impulse had been right. It had to be. If memory left no mark, then there could be no such thing as memory, no such thing as a personal past, no learning, no store of intimate and exotic knowledge. And if not that, then how to explain your sudden blinding reminiscence of that day in seventh grade when you dove headlong for the loose ball and crashed nose first into the bleachers and the pain was so sharp and bright you thought you had broken your brain, or the dense, long evening in the summer of the next year when you kissed Sharon Connelly, and she kissed back? If these things had truly happened, if you knew them to be true and had kept each in its own special place all that while, there was memory and it had only to be excavated from wherever it lay. Where was that place? What did it look like? Half a century after Lashley, no one knew.

Many of the experimental data marshaled from contemporary investigations of memory have been frail and indirect, some so slight that within the intimate, intensely competitive, and feud-ridden field of memory research, they are sarcastically dismissed as "investigator dependent," meaning they are derived from experiments done in particular labs but that no one outside those labs could replicate and few believed. Even the best of the data—that is, that which came from experiments that can be reliably duplicated—is often so narrowly focused as to be nearly useless in building larger explanations of how memories might be laid down.

The experiments—good and bad alike—used to generate all these results are, even when they work, seldom designed to test questions directly. They can't be. This is more than anything a reflection of the fundamental difficulty of neuroscience. Lashley failed not because he was wrong, but because he had no good way to look for his answer. The secrets are buried too deeply to be uncovered through direct observation. They literally can't be seen. The scale of the target environment—the brain—is forbidding. The three and one-half pounds of the average human brain are thought to contain something on the order of 100 billion neurons. The average neuron is far smaller than the thickness of a human hair, yet it contains many thousands of proteins, acting sometimes in unison, often in opposition, almost always in complicated combinations.

Almost all memory research—in Lashley's day as now—is done by implication. For most of human history, memory investigators have been forced to stand outside the brain, trying to determine what goes on in the lost world inside. The tools long did not exist to look directly for the answers to researchers' questions. Lynch was part of the generation of scientists that came after Lashley and for the first time moved the search into the complex machinery of the brain's interior. His generation has advanced to the threshold of addressing some of the great fundamental questions of the human condition. The move from outside in has finally given them a fighting chance to uncover the molecular mechanisms of the brain—to learn what actually happens when people think and talk, how they learn and remember.

PLAYING SCIENCE

That first day, my conversation with Lynch went something like this:

> ME: I'm interested in spending time in a laboratory, like yours, where the principal focus is the study of memory. I'd like to explain how memory functions and fails, and why, and use the work in the lab as a means to illustrate how we know what we know.
>
> LYNCH: You'd be welcome to come here. This would actually be a propitious time to be in the lab.
>
> ME: Why's that?
>
> LYNCH: Because we're about to nail this motherfucker to the door.

In the years after that meeting, I spent a great deal of time in Lynch's lab. I spoke with the other scientists and students who worked there and observed their experiments; I read papers they and others published; and I learned how to perform some of the most rudimentary tasks of their basic experiments. But what I mostly did at Lynch Lab was talk to Lynch. Or, rather, I listened as Lynch expounded on mammalian biology and brain science. This was a generous undertaking on his part, as I had arrived at the lab largely ignorant of the field. Listening to him often entailed following swooping, exhilarating flights over time and intellectual terrain. Bear with me, he sometimes said, this might not seem connected to what we've been talking about, but it will circle back. Ten, twenty, or thirty minutes later—often after side trips to Planck's constant, or Yankee Stadium, or Bismarck's Germany, or his childhood backyard in Delaware—it did.

Lynch almost always spoke in such a way that his huge ambition, self-regard, and lack of pretense were vividly displayed. He was unreserved, witty, juvenile, insightful, and learned in ways that were surprising. His conversation rippled with allusion. He was more apt to quote Cormac McCarthy than Charles Darwin. That first claim, that he was "about to nail this motherfucker to the door," was, in addition to being a status report on his research, a reference to Martin Luther (like Lynch, a conspirator against the establishment) nailing his indictment of the Roman Catholic Church to a cathedral door in sixteenth-century Germany. In subsequent talks, Lynch made similar on-the-fly references to, among many other things, left-handed relief pitchers, Moses, British naval history, the venture capital market, Kaiser Wilhelm II, Maxwell's equations, the ur-city of Ur, Dylan, Kant, Chomsky, Bush, Tacitus (whom he compared, unfavorably, to Suetonius), Titian, field theory, drag racing, his father's perpetual habit of calling him (intentionally) by the wrong name, his career as a gas jockey at an all-night service station, Pickett's charge at Gettysburg, Caesar's crossing of the Rubicon, and the search for the historical Jesus.

He was no less prolix in more formal settings. Eniko Kramar, a senior scientist in Lynch's lab, recounted a talk he had given to a conference on schizophrenia. Lynch outlined an emerging hypothesis based mainly on novel experiments then being conducted in the lab, but his talk ranged all the way back to his graduate school studies at Princeton. He even showed a slide, without identifying its origin, from his 1968 dissertation. Besides the fact that work he had done thirty-five years earlier was still relevant, Kramar said, "the sweep and elegance of it was breathtaking."

Lynch had moved his lab and office numerous times during his Irvine career, often as the result of some perceived, or real, slight. For a while his office was just a desk at the end of a communal hallway. The current lab was at 101 Theory Drive, in a tilt-up office park between a toll road and the University of California, Irvine, main campus. Lynch had ended up in the office park largely because everyone, including him, had concluded that all parties would be better served if there were some physical distance between Lynch and his university peers.

The university had put up the low-rise buildings in the 1990s in partnership with a developer, intending them to become a research nexus where academic and entrepreneurial talent could mix. It hadn't quite worked out that way. The rents were so high few truly innovative companies could afford the space. Most of the tenants had little if anything to do with the university. En route to the office park's resident Starbucks, Lynch often trailed whole convoys of shirttailed, triple-shot-latte addicts who spent their days and nights writing World of Warcraft code. That their dense, imaginary world was next door to a lab of neurophysiologists cutting up rat brains was utterly unknown to them. None of the work in the lab was apparent from the outside. The beige-on-beige, spray-on stucco building was indistinguishable from those in front of, beside, and behind it. More than once I walked into the wrong lobby.

The lab's address on Theory Drive was a developer's idea of a scientific street name. (The next left down the main road is Innovation Drive.) Lynch finds the name embarrassing. A kind of lunch-bucket anti-intellectualism prevails in academic biology, and Lynch was sometimes seen as guilty of its gravest sin— ambition. He mocks the criticism: " 'Oh a theory, another theory. That's cute. Look, guys, Gary has another theory.' " For all his bombast and the resentments it provoked, Lynch was not eager to antagonize his many enemies heedlessly. He was respectful of the intellectual protocols that placed formal biological theory on a very high shelf he had yet to reach.

It is a mark of the difficulty of the life sciences—biology and its many complicated derivatives—that to call something a theory is not to slight but to honor it. Theory, the developmental biologist P. Z. Myers has written, is what biologists aspire to. Scattered across the globe, more than a dozen places proudly proclaim themselves home to the pursuit of theoretical physics. But as Lynch notes, it is no accident that there is "no Institute for Neuroscience Theory." His protestations aside, he was almost constantly struggling for higher explanations, to make things cohere, to fit data into what the analytical philosopher Willard V. O. Quine called the web of science. In any event, insofar as the street was concerned, Lynch said, "I would have called it Hypothesis Drive."

Hypotheses and theories, while related, are more different than alike. The hypothesis is the fundamental organizing principle in scientific research. Its "if this, then that" structure underlies almost all scientific investigation. *If* is the key word in that construction. An hypothesis is a set of questions. A theory is a set of proposed answers.

Imagine the brain as a huge storehouse with shelf after shelf, miles long, filled with a wild assortment of tableware—teacups, saucers, platters, ceramic bowls, crude pottery, fine china, simple dinner plates. The tableware may once have been stored tidily, but an earthquake has leveled the interior. The resulting huge pile of wrecked shelves and broken plates is the geography that a neuroscientist must navigate while trying to discern patterns and coherence in the brain.

An hypothesis is what someone, after surveying the wreckage of that pile of plates, might offer to begin putting the pieces back together. If all the blue pieces go together, then maybe we can rebuild the bowls. Frequently—always, really—the view of the pile inside the brain is incomplete. Pieces big and small are missing. Sometimes they sit out of sight for decades, even centuries, with no one willing or able to imagine their having a place in the reconstructed order. Perhaps they're obscured by other pieces, or in another room, or lying in plain sight but are the wrong color. Who could possibly have imagined that brown shard would fit between the two blue? Lynch's true gift is an ability to see how varied pieces might fit together, to intuit that somewhere in the room—under that blue-black pile, perhaps—there ought to be a piece of green ceramic.

For thirty years the work in Lynch Lab has been driven by a single inquiry: What happens in the brain when a human being encounters a new experience such that he or she in the future—tonight, tomorrow, in the year 2025—can recall it at will? For much of that same amount of time, Lynch's efforts to answer that question have been governed by a single overarching hypothesis: If a process called long-term potentiation (LTP) is the means by which memory is encoded, and if memory is to be long-lasting, then brain cells have to change shape during LTP, and networks of these cells with altered shapes are the underpinning of memory.

The details of the biochemical interactions that cause the shape-changing, Lynch acknowledged, are enormously complex and not well understood. At the time he originally proposed it, in fact, they were not understood at all. But the crux of his hypothesis is that human interaction with the environment results in an actual physical change in specified cells in specified places in the brain and that those changed structures are permanent and form the component parts (what scientists call the substrate) of memory. Such rapid structural change is rare in biology of any sort. It just doesn't happen much anywhere, and there was very little evidence it happened at all in the mammalian brain.

Lynch now thought he was close to knowing how such a quick-change mechanism might work—or at least close enough to know if the path he had been pursuing all these years would eventually lead to answers or to a dead end. Science is shot through with just such failures; one more dead hypothesis wouldn't be widely noted. For Lynch, such an outcome would mean not simply a failed experiment but a wasted career.

It happens more than one likes to contemplate. Innumerable scientists, very good, even brilliant scientists, have poured the whole of their careers into pursuits that bring their brilliance up short, that yield little but frustration. Think of Lashley's search for the engram. A biologist once told me that he had spent 99 percent of his life searching for, and failing to find, a single molecule. Ninety-nine percent! The other 1 percent, he said, was breathing. It is often said that such nominally unsuccessful work produces as much knowledge as experiments that go as planned. Certainly learning what isn't true is useful information, but Nobel Prizes are not awarded for null experiments.

One way or another, Lynch, by the time I arrived in his lab, was certain he was near to finding out on which end of the scale he had laid himself. He was then sixty-one years old. I knew that he had been an often-polarizing figure in the field, that he had a reputation for being exceptionally, even stupidly, pugnacious, but also that he had been uncannily right about a lot of things over a very long time. This combination of success and belligerence produced a complicated legacy. In public, neuroscientists don't denigrate one another—or even disagree—a great deal. In private, they are world-class scoffers and backstabbers. Despite his clear accomplishments, no neuroscientist had been scoffed at more than Lynch.

Theo Wallimann, a biologist at ETH Zurich, has written: "Science and innovation are chaotic, stochastic processes that cannot be governed and controlled by desk-bound planners and politicians, whatever their intentions. Good scientists are by definition anarchists." Lynch fits the mode exactly.

Richard Thompson, a renowned neuropsychologist at the

University of Southern California, told me he had more than once nominated Lynch to membership in the prestigious National Academy of Sciences, only to be told by other members that Lynch would not be elected so long as they drew breath. By way of explanation, Thompson said: "There's a reason for his paranoia. There are a lot of people out there who don't like him. Gary doesn't suffer fools gladly." He paused, then chuckled. "And there are a lot of fools in the world."

However low the regard in which he was held, Lynch had slogged along, making hard and, considered collectively, astonishing progress, documented in more than six hundred published papers, some of which are now considered classics in the field and among the most frequently cited works in all of neuroscience. Lynch had succeeded, insofar as he had, by perseverance and by somehow intuiting, if not the answers to all his questions, at least a sense of where the answers might be found and what they ought to look like.

Notably among neuroscientists, Lynch crosses disciplines at will, moving from biochemistry to physiology to computer network modeling. "There are very few people who can do this. They're rare," said Richard Morris, one of England's most prominent neuroscientists.

Christine Gall, Lynch's frequent collaborator and longtime significant other, said: "Gary just has more RAM than other people. He can access lateral information that most people can't. It isn't like he has to think and remind himself. It's right there. He has access to it. He'll say, 'There's this,' and you'll say, 'Well, I knew that.' Except for you it has gone back into the archives and you don't think to make the link. To have that available to inform you, to make the next cognitive leap, that's his strength."

That leaping ability often led Lynch to situations in which he would say of an experiment: "This will never work. It can't." Then he would say: "But it has to." It has also earned him as much trouble as reward. He has never shied from making proclamations based on his intuitions, or from criticizing those not privy to his insight. "That is what amazes me," he says.

> People will walk in who are very sensible and intelligent biologists and tell you, "Memory is this." And you go, "How in the fuck could it possibly be that? I didn't think it was that when I was back at Our Lady of Fatima Grade School. I mean, I didn't think it was that when I was working at the all-night gas station. FOR CRYING OUT LOUD!"

One result of this perhaps excessive straightforwardness has been a more or less constant war with much of the neuroscience establishment, with university administrators, and with colleagues at Irvine. He jokes about this ruefully: "It would have killed a lesser man."

For much of its history, the search for an understanding of mental processes, including memory, has been primarily an intellectual adventure. It was first taken up by theologians and magicians, then philosophers, and, finally, scientists seeking understanding for its own sake. That has changed. Exploration of the brain is no longer a mere academic pursuit. Scientific interest in memory has never been greater than now, because, in addition to the development of tools to better ask questions about it, there is a more pressing need to learn the answers. Medical advances allow more people to live longer each year but have been unable to relieve longevity of its principal bane: the breakdown of mental processes, including especially memory— which, when it occurs, seldom fails to impress upon its victims and those who know them the extent to which our memories constitute our selves.

We are in the midst of a dementia pandemic. An estimated 6 million Americans have Alzheimer's disease today. That number has been growing exponentially; ironically, as medical care improves and people live longer each decade, it will continue to do so. Alzheimer's is just one of many neurodegenerative diseases whose incidence is increasing. By the year 2050 an estimated 100 million people worldwide will suffer from it or from Huntington's, Parkinson's, severe depression, or other dementias. The cost of treating these diseases goes up as well and will multiply as the population ages. In 2009 Alzheimer's care alone cost Medicare an estimated $160 billion. By 2035 it could overtake the defense budget. At current rates of expansion, by 2050 Alzheimer's disease all by itself will cost Medicare more than $1 trillion annually.

Given the grim facts, a sense of tragedy looms as science has been able to do precious little to combat neural disorders. One reason for this failure has been our meager understanding of the cognitive processes that are crippled in the course of the diseases. This has not been for lack of effort. Thousands of scientists have spent careers and billions of dollars seeking and largely failing to unearth these secrets. Sadly, because science has not developed more thorough understandings of how the physical processes of learning and memory are supposed to work, there has been little that could be done to fix those processes when they break.

As a corollary to his research into basic memory mechanisms, Lynch has investigated means to alter the functioning of those mechanisms—that is, to develop a way to counter the various afflictions that erode the brain's abilities. Working with the chemist Gary Rogers, he invented a class of drugs, called ampakines, that, if they work, will not only improve memory but make the brain perform better in numerous other ways. Ampakines will, in theory, help restore the cognitive abilities lost with the debilities of old age. Drugs of this sort (called cognitive enhancers or simply smart pills) have been sought for a century.

Like much contemporary drug research, ampakine development had been slow going, but by the time of my first meeting with Lynch in 2004, the FDA was considering versions of his drugs for clinical trials, to determine whether their substantial promise could be fulfilled. Success would be a signal moment in neuroscience history. By chance, the ampakine drug trials, which were to be conducted independently of Lynch, would get under way just as the memory-mechanism research in his lab seemed headed toward its own finale. The convergence of these two lines of research—one practical, one purely theoretical—is rare. Lynch had a sense that answers he had spent a career chasing were at hand.

That both the lab research and the drug project seemed headed toward conclusions simultaneously left Lynch alternately eager at the opportunity and utterly despondent at the likelihood of failure. He knew, as every research scientist does, that almost everything almost always goes wrong. If, over time, science can be viewed as the steady extinction of ignorance, in the near term, in most labs on most days, ignorance wins hands down. That scientists can nonetheless generally be described as optimistic tells us that these supposedly hyperrational people are the real hopeless romantics among us.

Lynch is more romantic, and hopeless, than most.

If, in biology, a hypothesis holds for a while, surviving challenge and criticism, much of it improbably hostile, it may eventually come to some rough, general acceptance and may then be joined to other hypotheses to form something more far-reaching. Lynch's hypothesis of quick, structural change had reached this point. Neuroscientists habitually use a particular word to categorize such a body of thought—or collected wisdom—in a part of their science. They don't, as a layman might, refer to such a collection as a *theory*. Instead, they call it a *story*. After thirty years spent telling it, Lynch was perilously close to believing he knew the story of human memory—why it exists, how it works, how it fails. He was standing at a threshold of genuine discovery.

How often, he asked, has that ever happened in the history of neuroscience?

His lab's new technique promised to answer what had long been supposition, to validate his life's work, and to do so in such a way that you would literally see the result. There were days he could barely stand the anticipation.

Lynch was not always bombastic. Like a warrior resting after the fight, he could be wistful. "It's hard, too," he'd say, and shake his head, "when you're alone all these years, in a battle with fate, which is mean and juvenile." Then he'd pause, reflect on his possible pomposity, and say: "Come on, it's vanity. It's just pure vanity. It's the strangest mixture. If you're good, if you're any good at all, you put yourself in a situation where reality could come around and—WHACK!—knock you down. That's what you really are afraid of. If you don't have that, you're not playing science."

He was definitely playing science now. With the drug research and the approaching end to his three-decade journey through what he once characterized as a gulag of unyielding biology, he had a rare opportunity—a shot on goal, he called it.

"Come to the lab," he said. "This could get interesting."

CHAPTER TWO

Seeing

BUTTERFLIES OF THE SOUL

Who you are consists largely of two sets of inputs: your genes and your memories. You come into this world with the genes, a biochemical plan within each cell for how you will grow, mature, and, to a significant extent, age. Much of this basic plan is immutable. You can no more change your likelihood of developing male pattern baldness than you can change your maternal grandmother. What keeps this genetic plan from being wholly inexorable, however, is your ability to change, to learn, to adapt. Learning is the process by which memories are made, meaning that memory, far more than being a simple repository, is the principal shaper of who you are. This leads to obvious questions: What is this thing that makes us who we are? What happens inside your head when you park your car and walk to your office, a restaurant, or home? Who was your third-grade teacher? What was Euclid's third axiom? How do you know, when you want to drive it again, where your car is?

Most of the time, when people attempt to define memory, they speak in metaphors, drawing analogies between memories and filing cabinets, or photographs, or videotape replays. They might talk about what memories mean and what the loss of them portends. They almost never talk about what memories actually are. Why? The simplest answer is they do not know.

In one sense, of course, that assertion is ridiculous. We all know exactly what memories are. They are recollected pieces of the past. But that definition is at best partial, confining itself to the result and ignoring the process. The recollection—the memory brought to mind—is the psychological portion of it, the ideas, feelings, emotions that are brought back to awareness. Yet the fact is, memories are also physical entities. They are real things in the real world.

When pressed to describe them, however, even accomplished brain scientists can say very little with certainty. They're in there, in the brain, somewhere; they have to be. If you or I can recall it, there must be an "it" to be recalled. Memory is, has to be, a physical thing, a product of brain functions.

Sadly, however, the brain contains no tape for us to rewind—it contains instead 100 billion neurons, and memories are networks of neurons, hastily assembled and stored away, sometimes for seconds (just long enough to dial a telephone number) and sometimes for decades (long enough that you can recall the smell of your mother's apple pie as it cooled on the kitchen counter in August 1963).

Saying that memories are networks of neurons was about as far as anyone was prepared to go in the 1970s when Lynch entered the field of memory research. To have defined memories in such a vague way doesn't seem a huge accomplishment, but in fact even this was a considerable success achieved over a very long time.

Memory as a subject of inquiry and wonder is as old as humanity. Given memory's central role in any definition of self, it is not long after you discover that you are that you wonder who and how you are. You do not, if the historical record is an accurate indication, necessarily think that the first place you ought to look is that three-pound lump of gray-and-white matter between your ears. The ancients looked instead to those places they thought most vital to life. The Egyptians developed elaborate procedures for preserving the human body after death. They separated certain organs—the liver, for example—for preservation and after embalmment carefully put the heart back in with the mummy. They believed in reincarnation and thought the heart would be necessary in that next life. They tossed the brain in the trash.

The ancient Greeks were the first to hypothesize that the brain is the place where mental activities occur, but not until the seventeenth century would the brain become the more or less agreed-upon center of cognition and, with that, memory. René Descartes was probably the first to suggest a specific locale in the brain for memory—the pineal gland.

Beyond speculation, however, little was learned about mental activity in the thousand-plus years between the Greeks and Descartes. For much of that time, mental processes were not considered a subject of inquiry in the natural sciences. They were instead dispatched (consigned? elevated?) to the realms of religion and then philosophy, which regarded the brain from its exterior. Even after the brain became the consensus location of mental activity, few thought that activity originated in the brain's physical materials. Descartes settled on the view that humans had a dual nature: the physical apparatus of the body, and a "life force" originating in some ephemeral place called the mind that moved the body to action. This dualism has had a predominant place in theories of the brain ever since, and the nature of Cartesian "life forces" is vigorously debated to this day.

As physical science progressed and uncovered more of the body's most intimate anatomy, elaborate schemes were devised to tie the observed physical structures to the unobservable forces that presumably guided their actions. A recurring notion proposed that the nerves, which were shown in the laboratory to activate muscles, were more or less hollow tubes that operated by means of an hydraulic apparatus; the mind sent a liquid or gas (depending on who was doing the describing) out through the nerves, inflating the muscles.

Finally, in the late eighteenth century, the Italian physician Luigi Galvani ran electricity through the leg of a dead frog and produced a kick reaction identical to a kick that the frog would have produced if alive. He claimed that the life force was electrical in nature. His student Alessandro Volta proved that the electricity was carried not by a liquid (as Galvani supposed) but by a current, as normal electricity was. The device he constructed to test his hypothesis was the world's first battery.

A few decades later the Danish scientist Hans Christian Oersted was conducting a classroom demonstration using one of Volta's batteries when he noticed that if a wire was connected to the two poles of the battery, the needle on a nearby compass moved. Oersted had accidentally discovered that magnetism and electricity were united, and in the process he had discovered a tool (what we call a volt meter) to measure electric current. In the mid-nineteenth century Emil du Bois-Reymond, a German physiologist, was among the first to attach such a device to a nerve. When he did, the needle jumped, meaning there was current in the animal nerve. "If I do not greatly deceive myself," he wrote, "I have succeeded in realizing . . . the hundred years' dream of physicists and physiologists, to wit, the identification of the nervous principle with electricity." Further research determined that the speed of the electric current through the nerve is on average about 27 meters per second, fast (the hundred-yard dash in under three seconds) but nowhere near lightning fast.

In the same period other scientists—notably Theodor Schwann and Matthias Jakob Schleiden—were working out what eventually became known as Cell Theory, which posits that all life-forms are made up of individual cells and that the cells in all organisms are more or less the same; complicated animals simply have more of them and more connections among them. This huge conceptual achievement is in many ways the central insight in the history of modern biological science, the infrastructure upon which Charles Darwin and Alfred Russel Wallace erected the theory of evolution. Yet for decades afterward scientists held that somehow the human brain was—of all living things in the living world—the sole exception.

At the end of the century a Spanish anatomist shattered that myth with a series of exquisite experiments that resulted in the first detailed images of individual neurons. Santiago Ramón y Cajal used a new staining technique to demonstrate that individual neurons are distinct from one another. Cajal showed that, contrary to belief and desire, the human brain, much like all other living organisms, is built out of individual cells enmeshed in a web of connections. In hypothesizing this Neuron Doctrine, Cajal powerfully imported the Cell Theory to the brain.

The staining technique allowed Cajal to view the neuron as a single entity, which he then determined has three main components: the main cell body; a single extension of the cell that he named the axon; and more numerous extensions that he called dendrites (derived from the Greek for *tree*). Both the axon and the dendrites have extensive branching systems of their own. You might visualize a neuron as a tree; the trunk represents the cell body, the axon its roots, and the dendrites its branches.

Previous researchers had seen these features but could not make out which parts were attached to the others or, more problematically, whether they were interconnected. It was commonly thought that the nervous system was one continuous structure. The billions of neural cells were packed so tightly, it was impossible for researchers with early light microscopes even to see spaces between them. Those spaces are indeed exceptionally small—on average, the gap between neurons is about 20 nanometers (that is, 20 billionths of a meter; for reference, a human hair is about two thousand times as wide). The notion that the structure was some sort of hydraulic system had been discarded, yet the idea that the system somehow allowed substances to flow through the body was still the majority view. The substance had been switched from a liquid to electricity, but the metaphor remained.

It is easy to see why. Imagine flying over a vast, sprawling, thick forest from a mile above. You will see trees, but you will not be able to tell where one tree ends and the next begins. You will simply see a dense field of green. It would be natural for you to regard the forest as a single entity, as most scientists prior to Cajal indeed had done. The stain Cajal used randomly marked individual neurons while leaving the rest untouched. Since each stained neuron stood in sharp relief to those surrounding it, he was finally able to see them as individual entities, not directly connected to one another.

More than just making the unseen visible, Cajal hypothesized, correctly, the functional roles the observed anatomy implied. He proposed that the electric current du Bois-Reymond

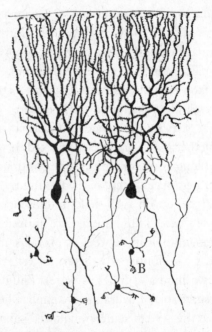

One of Cajal's drawings; it depicts two neurons.
(Courtesy of Larry Swanson)

had discovered ran through neurons in a systematic way, always moving from the dendrites through the cell body to the axon, then on to the dendrites of other neurons, beginning the cycle all over again. Because the axons and dendrites have extensive branches, each neuron is able to make contact with many others, potentially thousands. Cajal thought the axons met the dendrites at specific locations that Charles Sherrington would later call synapses. Neurons are contiguous but not continuous. Somehow the signal moves across the slightest gap between them. Nobel laureate Eric Kandel has likened this to whispering in someone's ear—moving close enough to be heard, but not to actually touch.

One powerful, practical insight Cajal derived from his studies was that the signals between neurons build networks that might be the underpinnings of memory. He proposed that the connections between neurons might, like muscles, be strengthened with use. Memory might be built out of mere brain matter. Cajal was searching for more than mere cellular connections: within them, he wrote, were hidden the greatest secrets of the self. He was hunting, he said, "the butterflies of the soul."

Cajal's discoveries and his careful, fastidious, irrefutable presentations (his drawings are still included in neuroscience textbooks) posed the questions that have consumed much of brain science since: How do neurons communicate with one another? How are they networked together? And how does the tremendous computational power of the brain arise out of those connections and communications?

TWENTIETH-CENTURY ADVANCES

Science to this day has a bare understanding of even the most primitive cells, each one of which, in the description of the English biologist Nick Lane, is "a minute universe." This is true of the humblest of cells and of the most complex. All are nano-worlds unto themselves, full of overflowing populations of protein molecules and tiny, intricate machines, some of them thousands of atoms long. So much activity in so small a place.

Each living cell has a semipermeable membrane encompassing a gelatinous interior that is studded throughout with various strange and tiny and largely unseeable structures. As you move from single-celled bacteria up through the orders of living things, the cells get far larger, from a few microns (millionths of a meter) in diameter to several thousand times bigger. And they are markedly more complicated. Cells in more advanced organisms have both more structures and more complex structures in their interiors, including a cell nucleus housing the organism's genetic instructions. They are also vastly more numerous. By the time mammals arrived (about 200 million years ago), organisms comprised billions upon billions of cells. Humans, it is estimated, have more than 50 trillion.

Cells in complex organisms, reflecting their origins in single-celled creatures, are in many respects self-sufficient. They contain much of the equipment necessary to sustain themselves and to manufacture their nutriment. Cells must also have a means to communicate with other cells. Without such signaling ability, a cell is little more than a bag of viscous fluid. Imagine the chaos in a factory in which workers couldn't communicate with one another. Nothing would ever roll off the assembly line.

Normal cells communicate primarily by exchanging proteins with one another and with the extracellular space between them. Different proteins pass from a cell to its neighbors or through the bloodstream to a distant location. (The latter frequent flier proteins are often referred to as hormones.) All cells have passageways through their membranes. Like gates in an ancient city wall, they are guarded and opened only to proteins that possess the proper credentials. Most proteins cannot pass through most gates, but if the right protein has the right identification, the gate opens wide, allowing the protein in. Nor do they just slink in and disappear into the city; once inside, they often start a wild party.

A neuron is a special kind of mammalian cell, differing by location, complexity, and means of communication. In the march from unicellular amoeba to man, the neuron arrived early—in jellyfish about 600 million years ago. This is a very long time, about 5 percent of the entire history of the universe and plenty long enough for evolution to have altered the neuron. Those in humans are markedly different from those in the earliest organisms, although the human neuron remains something of a black box, its internal workings still a mystery.

In humans every neuron contains approximately forty thousand proteins. Nobody has any idea what most of them are there for. A few of them have been singled out for study, but that is as much a matter of accidental discovery as scientific intent. They've been identified, therefore they get examined. Even if it were possible to know what each protein is, determining how they interact and what actions result from their interactions would be a forbidding undertaking.

What is clear is that over the eons the sheer number of neurons has multiplied and that neuronal interrelationships (and thus the systems constructed of them) have become more complex. A simple roundworm has about 300 neurons. A fruit fly has 300,000, and an octopus 30 million. You have, more or less, 100 billion. Size matters. The biggest difference between you and that worm (give or take a couple of arms, legs, and a backbone) lies mainly in those 99.999 billion extra neurons. That difference makes possible sophisticated cognition, memory, and consciousness, which is to say, you. The roundworm can't read, write, do brain surgery, or contemplate its mortality. There are no fruit fly Homers, no octopus Hamlets. David Foster Wallace famously considered the lobster. The lobster did not consider him.

In humans more than half of each individual's genes are directed solely to regulating the brain, which consumes a fifth of the energy produced by the body. Doing precisely what? we might ask. Cells in different parts of an organism share some traits with all of the organism's other cells, but they are almost always dedicated to specific functions. Cells in the liver digest and filter the fluids that pass through. Neurons send and receive signals. They have no other reason to exist. They do so by a method that was first outlined by Cajal but is far more complicated, almost comically so, than he imagined.

The basic signaling between neurons begins with a tiny spike of electricity called an action potential. For decades after du Bois-Reymond discovered this electric current, no one had any idea what caused it or exactly how it traveled through and across neurons. There were no wires to conduct this current through the brain. How did it move?

Alan Hodgkin, Andrew Huxley, and Bernard Katz unraveled the details in a series of papers in the early twentieth century. They used the squid as their experimental animal, because it has a very simple neural system and its individual parts are much larger and easier to identify than those in mammals. They hoped that the principles, once established in invertebrates, would also prove true in mammals, including humans.

Hodgkin, Huxley, Katz, and others eventually determined the means by which the current (which is small, about 100 millivolts, or a tenth of a volt; by comparison, a typical AA battery puts out about 1.5 volts) moves. If you recall basic high school chemistry, you know that some atoms carry electrical charges. These are called ions. It so happens that there are a great many more positively charged ions outside a neuron than inside. The difference between the inside and the outside is 70 millivolts. This is called the resting potential of the neuron.

Much of the energy the brain consumes is used to maintain this balance; potassium and sodium ions are constantly being pumped in and out of neurons. It seems mindless, and of course it is, which is to say it's undirected. But it is not purposeless. The intracellular negative balance must be maintained at a more or less constant level so that it can react uniformly to outside influences. Many of those influences arrive in the form of sensory inputs, themselves the results of interactions with the environment.

Here's an example of how such interactions happen. Let's suppose I want to go shopping at a shopping mall. I live in Cali-

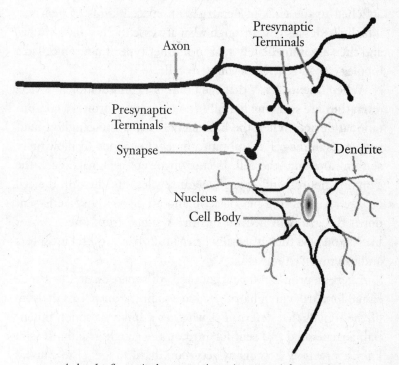

A sketch of a typical neuron. An action potential moves in the direction of the arrow down the axon to the synapse. Although it is not apparent from this highly simplified sketch, any one neuron is capable of forming multiple synapses with other neurons. In total, any one neuron might form thousands of synapses. (Courtesy of Lulu Y. Chen)

fornia, where most of the malls, including the one I'm turning into at the moment, are surrounded by huge expanses of parking lot. I travel up and down the parking aisles looking for a spot. I finally find one and pull in. It's a tight fit. The vehicle in the next spot is a huge SUV, a Hummer, making it nearly impossible for me to squeeze out of my door. My eyes—probably unconsciously—survey the parking lot. When the image of anything, for example the Hummer, enters my field of vision, it activates visual receptors called rods and cones, likely hundreds of them, on the retinas at the back of my eyes. Those receptors are attached to the ends of dendrites on special kinds of neurons. The light signals pass through what are essentially relay switches and then are immediately sent to another type of neuron called a bipolar cell and then to a ganglion cell.

When scientists say that the brain is a computational device, often they are speaking literally. In fact, each neuron is a computational device. When the light signals reach the ganglion neuron, gates in the cell membrane immediately open to allow more sodium ions into the cell. If enough receptor signals reach the ganglion neuron and enough sodium is let into the cell, the cell charge changes to a net positive and an electrical spike is sent down the ganglion neuron's axon. A signal from one receptor likely won't do this. It usually takes input from several receptors and can involve thousands.

Every neuron can form thousands of synapses, and to send a signal forward, enough of them have to fire at once. It is the sum of the signals that determines whether a spike, or action potential, is generated and sent forward on the ganglion axon. It isn't known precisely how many receptors have to signal to cause a spike, and the number changes depending on the specific environment, but something on the order of six to eight receptors seems to be a minimum. The spike is an all-or-nothing event. Its strength doesn't vary. Either the threshold is reached and a spike is sent, or it is not reached and nothing happens. This is true of all neural signals. If there is no spike, then even though your eyes received the initial light signal, you will not become aware of it.

The axons from the eye are bound together as they leave the eye, in a bundle of 1.5 million axons commonly known as the optic nerve. All information that leaves the eye destined for the brain travels on one of the axons in that bundle. Once the spike is sent, the ganglion gates close to the positively charged sodium ions and open to allow more negatively charged potassium back in, and the negative charge, the resting potential, is restored, awaiting the next batch of signals.

Meanwhile, the visual information about the parking spot I saw is zipping through my brain. Like all sensory signals sent to the brain, the visual information makes several stops before it gets to where it is eventually going. The axons of the optic nerve mainly end in a portion of the brain called the thalamus, an elaborate kind of switching station that sends the signals on through relays in other parts of the brain before reaching their final destination, the cortex. At each step axons relay the information to the dendrites of another set of neurons.

Recall that this whole process began when I was in the parking lot and particles of light struck my retina. These images were then converted to electrical signals and sent forward. Obviously, the interior of the brain is not exactly bathed with light. It is in almost every way a very dark place. Where the axons of the optic nerve end, there are no light particles to restart the process. How does the signal get relayed to the next neuron?

A remarkable thing happens. When the signal reaches the end of the axon, it causes tiny packages of chemicals to be released into the extracellular space. Specifically, they're released into the synaptic cleft, a very, very narrow space between the axon terminal and a dendrite of another cell. The chemical packages are filled with neurotransmitters, which drift across the cleft. Some of them fall onto receptors specially designed to receive them; others drift away. Those that bind to receptors do exactly what the light particles did at the beginning of the process—they cause channels to be opened into the dendrite that allow positively charged sodium ions into the cell.

This is happening simultaneously to perhaps thousands of different dendrites. Once again the receiving cell adds up the influx of sodium. If enough dendrites on the same neuron receive enough positively charged ions, the cell depolarizes (that is, becomes more positively charged), and a new spike is sent on to the cell nucleus and eventually onward down its axon. In effect, the original electrical signal is converted into a chemical signal, then reconverted back to electricity and sent on.

Not all of the neurotransmitter that is released into the synaptic cleft finds its way to a receptor. Some of it simply falls by the wayside. This is at best a curious construction, but in its own way it works. At each step the new set of neurons has to have enough inputs to cross the threshold for those neurons to spike and send a new action potential onward. If there is not enough signal, there is no spike; the information is lost. This happens routinely. The system is constructed so that loss of information is constant. Think about that for a minute. Your brain is wired to ensure that you routinely lose information, not because of some failing on your part but because it's built to do exactly that.

The neuron, remember, has been around for more than 600 million years. For more primitive animals, losing information might not matter. Frogs, for example, virtually never look at anything in their environment unless it is moving. You can put a frog in a room full of food, and if it is all frozen in place, the frog will starve to death. Fortunately for frogs, their food—flies, mosquitoes—is not frozen. It moves and gets eaten. The frog doesn't need an exact image of its surroundings. Humans use some of the same cognitive pieces as the frog.

Slightly higher on the evolutionary ladder, the reptilian brain is a large tangle of neurons comprising the brain stem (at the top of the spine) and the cerebellum (just behind it). Together they control the body movements required to stay alive—breathing and body temperature—and some broad motor responses. It is all the frog has. Early mammals add the limbic system, which controls automatic bodily functions such as digestion and blood pressure. The limbic system also includes new structures that help primitive brains record experience—the hippocampus and amygdala. They sit atop the reptilian brain. We have them too. Finally primates add the neocortex, the folds of gray matter that have grown in size to the point that, in humans, the neocortex by mass is about 80 percent of the brain. All three parts are wired together in a variety of what appear to be nearly random ways. Humans have, in effect, hijacked the frog's means of neural communication, the action potential, and plopped a cognition and memory machine on top of it.

David Linden, a neuroscientist at Johns Hopkins University in Baltimore, has likened the human brain to a three-scoop ice-cream cone. You get the frog's cognitive abilities on the bottom, maybe a squirrel in the middle, and *Homo sapiens* on top. A human brain is bigger than the frog's, with more parts and many more connections, but it retains some of the same limitations. For example, the speed of neural communication is the same in a human and in a frog. And while the frog's world has not changed dramatically since the first frogs, the world of humans has. This is a sharp reminder that natural evolution works at nothing close to the speed of human cultural evolution and technological innovation.

Even as biologists struggled throughout the twentieth century to discern and illuminate the microscale actions of individual neurons, they lacked a unified broader view of their subject. While they made slow, steady progress at the microscale of the cell, they made very little toward understanding how the brain works at higher levels. There was no generally accepted theory of the brain. A new field, psychology, rose to prominence trying to do precisely that, devising theories of the brain that would explain human behavior. Karl Lashley, although he failed to find an engram, was one of those engaged in this pursuit and to a significant extent legitimized it. The methods available in the first half of the twentieth century were notably crude. To try to correlate behavior with the brain, Lashley, and many others, used one main method: they removed portions of the brain, then looked to see what changed in the behavior of that particular brain's owner.

This method differs only in scale from the method used by the earliest molecular biologists to try to determine what effect a particular molecule might have in an organism. They would remove the molecule, then try to determine what was different in the organism. Lee Hartwell, a Nobel-laureate geneticist, has likened this technique to sitting in a car parked across the street from the main gate of a factory with tens of thousands of employees. Equipped only with a roster of who didn't come to work that day, the scientist was supposed to determine how the factory output was changed. The difficulty notwithstanding, plenty of scientists were willing to assume stakeout posts in those cold cars. In molecular biology, removing a gene was typically referred to as *ablating* it; the equivalent term in cognitive psychology was *lesioning*. So a typical experiment involved lesioning, or removing, a portion of the brain, then trying to determine what was missing in behavior. It was a blunt instrument, but few other tools were available.

The seminal event in the modern history of memory research was just such an operation that occurred more or less by accident in 1953. A young Connecticut man was having horrific epileptic seizures. In an effort to stop them, a highly regarded neurosurgeon named William Scoville removed a portion of the man's brain. The surgery stopped the seizures but also rendered the man (known in the literature as H.M.) incapable of forming new memories. The psychologist Brenda Milner examined H.M. over a period of months and determined that his memory of events from his childhood and adolescence were uninhibited. He simply could not make new memories. H.M. could readily learn to perform new tasks but by the next day would forget he had learned a task and had to relearn it. Scoville had removed sections of the temporal lobes, the areas just above and behind the ears. The main target of the surgery was a structure within the temporal lobes known as the hippocampus. The fact that after the hippocampus was removed H.M. could no longer form memories but could recall older ones suggested strongly that the hippocampus was crucial to making but not to storing memory. It immediately made the hippocampus the central focus of memory research.

Coincidentally, an ocean away in Norway, Per Andersen had spent years studying the hippocampus. Unlike Milner, a psychologist interested in the externally ascertainable effects of brain activity and injury, Andersen, a neurophysiologist, was not investigating memory. He was investigating how the brain works at the cellular level. He was methodically trying to build a basic understanding of the hippocampus's unique wiring system, which is much more ordered and systematic than that of other parts of the brain. Andersen routinely used pairs of slim glass electrodes, one to stimulate and one to record, to measure the passage of electric current through the hippocampus. He and others using the same method (called field recording) had long observed that bursts of relatively high-frequency electrical stimulation of particular pathways in the hippocampus produce a strong signal farther on in the pathway that persists for a short time after the stimulation has been applied. The effect was called potentiation.

In the early 1960s Terje Lomo came to Andersen's lab as a graduate student and began a more systematic investigation of the phenomenon. In 1964 he found that potentiation sometimes lasts for hours. As Andersen had before, Lomo put the result aside for several years to explore other aspects of the hippocampus and, not incidentally, to work on his Ph.D. dissertation. It wasn't until Tim Bliss, an English neuroscientist with a keen interest in malleability, or plasticity, as it was called, arrived in the lab four years later that Lomo returned to the subject. And even then, he worked on it only a day a week, in order to help Bliss. In the fall of 1969, Lomo and Bliss executed a version of Lomo's experiment in which they followed the effects of the initial high-frequency stimulation through the course of an entire night and were astonished to find the potentiation effect persisted.

In 1973 Bliss and Lomo published their first comprehensive paper on the effect they had discovered, which they called long-lasting potentiation. Bliss also published a follow-up paper with Tony Gardner-Medwin. Using a technique that Gardner-Medwin had developed, they determined that potentiation in living, unanesthetized animals lasts as long as thirty-six hours.

Potentiation in essence is an increase in the current passing between neurons. It seemed that the only way more current could be passed was to strengthen connections between neurons. Cajal had surmised seventy years earlier that the process of sending signals between neurons strengthens the bond between the sending and receiving cells, somewhat akin to the way repeated use makes muscles stronger. In other words, practice makes not perfect, but better; as the psychologist Donald Hebb put it, what fires together wires together. Lomo and Bliss seemed to give strong support to this long-standing hypothesis. Additionally, the combination of brief stimulation and long-lasting effect in the Bliss-Lomo experiments matched characteristics that scientists had long associated with memory.

Still, no one was all that excited about the findings, not even its discoverers, who quickly moved on to other lines of investigation. One reason the Bliss-Lomo discovery had little immediate impact was that it had no obvious application to the theory of memory dominant at the time, which held that memory formation occurs at the level of RNA, that is, in genetic materials. Since potentiation apparently did not involve changes in genetic material, many scientists downplayed its import. A second, and perhaps more powerful, reason was the simple fact that the Bliss-Lomo experiments were excruciatingly difficult to execute. Working with live animals made the experiments complicated and delicate. A precise surgery had to be done on every animal, to insert the stimulating and measuring electrodes into their brains. The measurements were often vague. A lot went wrong. Even Lomo and Bliss had a hard time repeating their own experiments.

One scholar later said their research was "not thought to be relevant to any outstanding problems, nor did it provide remarkable answers about the brain's structure or function. It was simply an interesting characteristic of a relatively unknown region of the brain." To be fair, the Oslo group within which most of this work occurred was interested mainly in mapping the wiring of the brain. The hippocampus was of little more interest than any other region, and there were plenty of other regions to map. As a laboratory phenomenon, long-lasting potentiation seemed interesting but not earthshaking.

The initial papers did not make large claims for the potentiation phenomenon; in fact, their claims were quite modest. The researchers wondered what sort of mechanism might cause the changes to persist but shied from discussing psychological implications. The most profound implication was that the potentiation effect seemed exactly the sort of process that psychologists had long hypothesized as the foundation of memory. It was generally agreed then that memory, as hypothesized as far back as the late nineteenth century, was somehow built out of networks of neurons. How those networks got built remained a central question of memory research when Gary Lynch arrived in Irvine in the fall of 1969.

CHAPTER THREE

A Strange Damn Place

THE FREE-RIDE GUY, 1960S

Gary Lynch was born the third of four children, the youngest son in a disintegrating Irish Catholic working-class family in a largely Italian Catholic neighborhood in Wilmington, Delaware. His father, known as Harry, was such an odd and often unfriendly man that Lynch claims still to not know his real name. Harry was a physical, foreboding presence who for reasons of his own never called Gary Lynch by his given name but used Mike as a substitute. As in *Goddammit, Mike, get over here,* or *Goddammit, Mike, you see that pitch?* Gary's older brothers were local toughs and in constant trouble; Gary became his mother's protector in increasingly intense disputes with his father. The parents eventually separated.

Gary seems to have shared at least two things with his father—an intense disregard for authority and a passionate love of baseball. More to the latter point, Lynch is not simply a baseball fan but, for reasons of birth and other ungovernable circumstance, a Philadelphia Phillies fan. If one were to know nothing else about Lynch but that he was a Phillies fan, one would know a lot. A baseball fan, as any baseball fan knows, lives in a state of dread and its always imminent companion, despair; the general outlook of a Phillies fan would have to improve markedly to reach despair. In 2007 the Phillies became the first professional team in the history of all team sports to lose ten thousand games. Granted, it took more than one hundred years, and they actually won the World Series the next year, but that is an awful lot of disappointment. As it happens, this is a perfect fit to brain science, which makes being a Phillies fan look almost like fun.

Lynch earned scholarships to Catholic high school, then the University of Delaware—"always a free-ride guy," he said. He had no expectations for college beyond the opportunities to meet girls and have fun. He went not because he had any inkling of what he wanted to learn or become, but because, for a bright kid without any obvious abilities, it was the expected and simplest path. He enrolled as an engineering major because a friend had told him it would be a good way to make a living. He subsequently was shocked to discover that a frighteningly small number of his fellow majors were women and that the budding engineers, after being tortured all week, returned, gladly it seemed, to their workshops on weekends to practice building electrical circuits.

Sitting amid unbathed teenaged boys wrapping wires around terminals was not Lynch's notion of collegiate life, and he was beginning to despair when fate intervened. After one particularly egregious episode among many involving too much alcohol and too much mouth, Lynch was kicked out of school for excessive partying. The free ride had ended abruptly; he was forced to work odd jobs, including a stint as a pump jockey at an all-night gas station, until he was readmitted. When he came back, he took art history classes; there were lots of girls, several of whom seemed to be majoring in psychology. He joined them. "It looked easy," he recalled. "I worked the angles, did the least amount of work I possibly could."

Lynch caught another break with the then-mandatory ROTC classes. He was a far-from-ideal soldier candidate, but as a boy he had had a keen interest in military history. Upon his return to school he enrolled in a required course that focused on the American Civil War, a subject that had obsessed him for years. The tradition at UD was that the top military history student would be honored at a spring ROTC convocation. The instructor realized that Lynch knew more about the Civil War than anyone in the class, even himself (correcting him, for instance, on where General James Longstreet's Confederate troops were positioned—badly, it turned out—on the second day of the Battle of Gettysburg), and there was no way he could legitimately keep Lynch from winning the award. Given Lynch's profound lack of military bearing, this would have been a genuine embarrassment. The ROTC command quickly made a deal absolving Lynch of all further ROTC obligations, in return for which he merely had to not compete for the award. He happily obliged.

Lynch, in spite of this professed laziness, prospered at UD. All the while, he thought, I'm great back here, but what happens when I get around a bunch of smart people? He found out soon after he earned a graduate scholarship to Princeton, where, he quickly determined, he would fare just fine. And for those interested in foreshadowing: on his first day on campus at Princeton, Lynch heard for the first time the Rolling Stones song "(I Can't Get No) Satisfaction."

While earning his graduate degrees in a remarkably brief time, he determined that psychology as a career would do little more than frustrate him. Psychologists stood outside the brain and asked questions about it and about its owner. They gave tests and made inferences—informed speculations, really—about what went on inside. "It's a tough job," he said. "It's just babbling, but at some level they have to try to explain everything. Well, they already did. Freud explained it all. Of course, it was total horseshit, but it explained everything."

Lynch realized he was much more interested in the emerging science of the brain's interior, what went on inside, and began plowing through the realms of flesh and blood and biology. "I got into the brain early in graduate school solely to get away from asking, 'Why do rats run on a wheel?' which was all anybody else seemed interested in doing," he said.

"Rats on a wheel" is his shorthand for behavioral psychology, which he had decided was more guesswork and wishes than true science. He had some company: in the 1950s and 1960s, scientists began the first broad, sustained effort to turn the study of the brain away from pure psychology. Sigmund Freud's theories of the psychological underpinnings of the human brain dominated current belief and practice, but scientists were frustrated by the theoretical and untestable nature of the ideas. Even those who agreed with Freud wanted to look into the brain and see where the Freudian id and ego were buried. They began to find and refine new tools that let them move inside the brain rather than simply observe it from without. Brain science was poised to become more investigation than observation.

Despite not having successfully navigated a biology course since high school—too many details, he said—Lynch taught himself neuroanatomy and as a grad student ended up teaching one of the first courses Princeton had ever offered on that subject. He earned his Ph.D. in psychology in 1968, just three years after enrolling. Soon afterward, he received a job offer from UC Irvine, of which he had barely heard. The university, just three years old, hadn't yet graduated its first class. The offer was to teach in the psychobiology department.

Lynch had no formal background in biology—none. He hadn't been to California—not once. But one of the first of those now-ubiquitous lists of the best universities had been recently published. For purposes of this ranking, UC Berkeley (which had no medical school) and UC San Francisco med school (which had no undergraduate program) had been combined and ranked number one among all universities in the world. "It's the fucking people's university," said Lynch. "That's a public university. Oxford, Cambridge are down here; Harvard's down here; Princeton's down here. The best university in the world is a public university. I thought, Man, we are so on the right track. That inspired me. I thought, This is it, this is finally it. In the face of people working on great things together in the sunshine, in the eternal summer of California, privilege falls away. What could be more beautiful?"

Not mentioned was the fact that California was broadly perceived to be the world headquarters of a cultural revolution Lynch was eager to join. He took the job. Orange County, where Irvine is located, was not, however, to be confused with Berkeley. It was nearly its opposite—politically conservative, headquarters to the ultraright John Birch Society, and decidedly not cosmopolitan. The city of Irvine had been designed not by city planners or architects or natural market actions but by a private development company. It was in almost every way an artificial construct and, at that, still largely theoretical. When Lynch arrived, the town was not far removed from its ranchland past. It was a mainly agricultural preserve, full of citrus groves and pastures. Cattle still grazed on the hills above the campus, and cowboys still chased them.

The physical surroundings might have been modest; the goals were anything but. The construction of the Irvine campus was part of one of the grandest, most ambitious academic undertakings in history. This was California in its golden age, California at its glorious best, systematically building an intellectual infrastructure unprecedented in the history of humankind. The state's higher-education budget had tripled between 1945 and 1955; then a new president, Clark Kerr, devised and won legislative approval for an even more ambitious expansion of the system, creating, in addition to Irvine, new universities at San Diego and Santa Cruz out of empty hilltops, seemingly overnight. California recruiters cruised through the academic world looking to hire away whole departments. The system expanded to ten campuses, including professional schools for medicine and law, even specialized schools of astronomy and oceanography. In the same period a system of state teachers' colleges began offering two-year degrees, then four, and, finally graduate degrees.

The University of California system was among the most remarkable achievements in a California century stuffed full of remarkable achievements. Nothing like it had ever been built in so short a time anywhere on earth. The development of so rich and vast an education system paired with the state's magnificent physical endowment to create a place where almost everything seemed possible.

Neuroscience, too, was young, and there was a sense broadly shared within it that the human brain, one of the last great frontiers of science, was about to be colonized, although from which direction or by whose army was unclear. Biologists, chemists, anatomists, physicians, psychologists, mathematicians, even philosophers and physicists, all suddenly calling themselves neuroscientists, plunged into the field. No one knew where they were going, and no one wanted to be left behind.

Lynch was just twenty-six when he arrived in Irvine in 1969, wild-eyed, bushy-haired, and bearded, fully a man of his time—perhaps a bit too fully. It was The Sixties, it was southern California in the Age of Aquarius, land of eternal light and equally endless good times. Lynch fit; he became a creature of the time and place. The university had been built more or less in the middle of nowhere, on the leeward side of striking sandstone bluffs, as the center of an ambitious real estate development a few miles inland from the Pacific Ocean. Only in California would a world center of brain science emerge as an adjunct to a sea of subdivisions.

Lynch moved into a permanent party pad at the beach on Balboa Island, a free-fire zone of drugs and bacchanalia. Never one to ignore a party, he reveled in the lifestyle. He remembers awakening on more than one morning after a party, "me and Sparky [Sam Deadwyler, a postdoc] driving to work with the windows down, still drunk, the car smelling like a brewery," singing along at the top of their lungs to The Who's "Won't Get Fooled Again." His apartment was outfitted with a mattress, a chair, and a telephone. "And," said a friend from those years, "he never answered the phone."

An unnerving number of people from the time describe bonding with Lynch in a bar. Given the era and his inclinations—he recounts regularly skipping out of scientific seminar ballrooms to fire up joints in the alley with other, now prominent scientists, some of whom wish his memory weren't so keen—this was perhaps a good thing. Bars at least were legal.

Given four hundred square feet of lab space and $900 to equip it ("I forgot to ask about money," he said about his employment negotiations), Lynch went to work. One of the hallmarks of his career has been that no matter how unruly a life he manages—or fails to manage—outside the lab, he is never outside it for long. He is a creature of the lab. To say he is driven would be understatement: he is possessed.

Very quickly, continuing work he had begun in grad school at Princeton, he made discoveries having to do with the brain's ability—a surprise at the time—to repair damage to itself after injury. It had generally been thought that the brain, especially the evolutionarily most advanced portion of it, the neocortex, was static, that it did not produce new cells or structures after it reached maturity. Lynch's discovery, and others made in the same period, posed a serious challenge to this view.

Lynch found that the cortex produces new synapses, literally "sprouts" them, after injury. This seemed unbelievable, not just to him but to many others. The brain just didn't do that. He repeated the experiments. They worked every time. Well, critics said, perhaps the sprouting occurs, but there is no way the new growth could actually produce functional connections in the brain. Lynch, working with UCI colleague Carl Cotman (who, Lynch said, was, unlike himself, supposed "to be a real scientist"), tested the functionality, and the initial results held up. The sprouting yielded functional new connections.

"This was a bombshell," Lynch marveled. "Sprouting was the thing that gave me this attitude that, 'Yeah, I know everybody says that can't be done, but they don't know what the fuck they were talking about.' People like me and Cotman had an arrogance. If I never learned anything else from the Princetonians, it was that arrogance is good."

For a young scientist, publishing a paper or two in decent journals during his first few years on faculty would be considered a good start to a promising academic career. In a single year, 1973, Lynch published a dozen papers on the sprouting phenomenon. He and Cotman became two of the hottest young guns in the neuroscience world. Irvine, under the leadership of Dick Thompson and Jim McGaugh, suddenly became a world center of brain research. Scientists who would go on to great renown congregated seemingly by accident; within a few short years they built one of the planet's premier neuroscience research facilities. A certain giddiness to the scene made it seem surreal. Anything could happen.

Just to follow the implications of the sprouting experiments, Lynch had to teach himself neurophysiology. A natural autodidact, he plunged into the literature. He had always taken a rare enjoyment in solitary contemplation, was happiest when sitting alone reading or immersed in data. (Understanding and reveling in statistics was the one great benefit of his formal education in psychology.) He and other researchers began to wonder if the brain did not possess more inherent plasticity than had been assumed. Perhaps structural change was a prevalent phenomenon in the normal, undamaged brain. If so, then the brain was a far different structure than had been imagined.

While Lynch was trying to figure out what exactly was going on with the sprouting, the Bliss-Lomo-Gardner papers were published. Lynch read them upon publication in the summer of

1973 while sitting in a university corridor waiting for a seminar to begin. He thought the researchers must have somehow stimulated a sprouting effect just as he had in his experiments, so he was immediately interested. "Otherwise, why would it last?" he wondered.

By sheer coincidence, the next day Lynch read a paper by a different group of scientists describing a technique they had invented for studying pathways in the brain. By placing very thin slices of the hippocampus in a nutrient- and oxygen-rich container to keep it sufficiently alive, they had been able to perform experiments, tracing the electrical circuits of the slice for hours after the hippocampus had been surgically removed from an animal. Although the paper was seven years old and the technique was a standard one in use with other tissues in biochemistry, Lynch found it utterly unbelievable that it would work with brain tissue. One of the difficulties of brain science was the lack of experimental techniques that did not require the use of live animals. This technique seemed too good to believe.

"Jesus Christ, there's something that can't be true," he said. "I thought it was absolutely impossible. Maybe it was just superstition. This was the brain! But if this was true, everybody in the world would be doing it. It's crazy. If it's true, you could do anything in the lab. You could combine chemistry, physiology, and anatomy in one shot."

Lynch at the time had not done any work on memory. As a casual observer, he was aghast that the gene theory of memory was being taken seriously by those in the field. Reputable scientists were training earthworms so that they would avoid being exposed to electric shocks, grinding up the worms and feeding the bits to other worms, then somehow ascertaining that the memories to avoid shocks were transferred from the eaten worms to the eaters. "It was insane," Lynch recalled thinking. "It could not be true."

He assumed that the potentiation effect was somehow related

to his sprouting work, so he set out to see if he could replicate the Bliss-Lomo experiments. He did, but he was wrong about what was causing the effect. "The first day I got a potentiation response, I knew it couldn't be sprouting," he said. "It happened too quickly." The sprouting phenomenon happened over the course of several days. The Bliss-Lomo effect happened immediately, in seconds. Lynch thought it was something utterly new, powerful, and important. He thought the best way to study it would be to use the slice technology he had just stumbled upon.

The normal course of action would have been to send a student or postdoc to the lab in England that had developed the technique, have that person learn it, and then bring it back to Irvine. Lynch didn't think he had time. The combination of the potentiation discovery and the slice technique was too powerful— everybody would jump on it, he thought. It would be a huge race, and he couldn't spare the time to get properly trained.

So he gave his lab the task of building brain slice chambers like those described in the paper. The scientists hacked something together pretty quickly so Lynch could see if the technique was even feasible. It was, but the lab had to redesign the chambers, which were far too complicated for day-to-day use. Consulting with Joe Biela, an engineer in UCI's machine shop, Lynch eventually settled on a design that consisted of a Plexiglas dish about the circumference of a regular lab petri dish, but taller, with cutouts in the lid through which electrodes could be inserted into the brain slice the dish contained. The electrodes were used in pairs—one to stimulate the tissue, the other to record the current that passed through the slice, which was submersed in a temperature-controlled, nutrient-rich liquid. Redesigning the chambers slowed progress, but so did Lynch's decision as to which area of the hippocampus to concentrate on.

One reason brain scientists love the hippocampus, apart from its presumed significance, is that it is largely a good neighborhood in which to work. It is, compared with much of the rest of the brain, orderly, neatly layered, and segregated; its circuitry is so clearly delineated, you can almost trace it with a pencil. It is well studied and well mapped; its regions are named with straightforward simplicity: CA1, CA3, and so on. If you choose to poke around there, you generally know what you are poking.

There is a place in the hippocampus, however, where the clarity and understanding run aground. It's called the dentate gyrus and is composed mainly of a peculiar type of neurons known as granule cells. These are generally thought to be the most primitive cells in the mammalian cortex. The dentate gyrus had no known function within the hippocampus's assumed, but still vague, role in memory formation. Yet there it was—"the strangest thing in the mammalian brain," Lynch called it.

The fact that it is located in what was thought to be the brain's memory center—in other words, in the middle of one of the most sophisticated structures ever evolved—bugged Lynch to no end. "There's no hypothesis," he said, so of course he set almost his entire lab to applying the new slice technique to study potentiation in granule cells in the dentate gyrus. "An awful, awful call," he said later.

Only one other research group had taken up the slice technique to study the potentiation effect. Oddly, it was Per Andersen's lab in Norway, where the original Lomo-Bliss experiments had been done. Andersen hadn't been at all interested in the work then. But when Bliss, Lomo, and Gardner-Medwin all went missing after they published their original papers, Andersen picked up where they left off. In adopting the slice method, he had a distinct advantage over Lynch. Where Lynch had had to teach himself brain anatomy, Andersen was a world-class physiologist and was much more adept than Lynch at navigating the hippocampus.

Lynch couldn't get anything to work. Even after he and his lab finally found a design for the slice chambers that allowed them to do the experiments he wanted, he struggled. For more than a year he tried to get the slice preparation to work in the dentate gyrus. That was where he had done his sprouting work, and even though he knew by then that the potentiation effect was distinct from sprouting, he persisted in trying to do the new experiments there.

It took more than two years to gather enough experimental results to publish a single paper. In the meantime another group published a paper referring to the Bliss-Lomo finding as "long-term potentiation," which was more in line with the previous nomenclature of memory research. Lynch adopted the new name and in talks and further publications popularized the acronym LTP, which became the standard method of referring to the phenomenon.

The early LTP literature studiously avoided implying that the work might have importance for the understanding of memory. People seldom even uttered the word *memory*. "You'd get your mouth washed out with soap if you did," Lynch said.

It was his willingness to see—even if heretically—the larger picture that gave Lynch whatever edge he might have over Andersen. He had a clear conception of where the potentiation work might lead. "Bliss vanished, Lomo vanished. Per picked up the slices with a couple of new postdocs. They did good work, but I think they had no idea what it was about," Lynch said. "For me, from the first minute I ever did an LTP experiment, I said, 'That's memory. That's fucking memory.' "

LYNCH LAB, 1970S

The duties of a university scientist heading his own lab are manifold. Foremost, the scientist—called the principal investigator, or PI—is the lab's intellectual leader, largely determining what research gets done. Graduate and postgraduate students come to labs not to bring new ideas to them but almost always to learn from the PI. Additionally, the PI does research, teaches, mentors, and presumably manages what amounts to a small business enterprise in an intensely competitive market niche. "It's all-consuming," said Tim Tully, a contemporary and sometimes competitor of Lynch who ran a lab for years at Cold Spring Harbor Laboratory in New York. "You can't do anything else. I'm not rested enough at the end of a day to read a paragraph, let alone a novel."

The existence of the lab depends on the PI's ability to fund it. He is an employee of the university but also a sort of profit center. He must attract grants, from which the university takes a significant cut (generally about one-third) as overhead, leaving the rest to pay the expenses of the laboratory—salaries, equipment, supplies, everything.

Although a handful of private foundations fund research, the overwhelming majority of grant money comes from the U.S. government; in the life sciences, most passes through the National Institutes of Health (NIH). NIH funding made possible the huge advances in biomedical knowledge achieved since World War II and fed the growth of academic science, multiplying the number of programs across the country. The growth was to an extent self-perpetuating—the more programs there were, the more scientists would be trained within them; the more scientists, the more applicants for the grant money.

The competition to receive money had become intense and bitter, and often left normally calm, civil-tongued scientists sounding like sailors with Tourette's syndrome: they went ballistic. Lynch, whose lab has been funded mostly by the federal government at around a million dollars per year for decades, is no exception. Hardly a day goes by in the lab without someone wondering aloud about getting or keeping a grant. In part because of this constant threat of extinction, neuroscience labs are not the happiest places on earth. There is tension and fear and jealousy and a near constant sense that careers are about to be made or missed. Such fraught situations call for careful, considered management.

Due to a lack of interest, or possibly ability, which can sometimes be the same thing, Lynch ran his lab like a young man on a midnight beer run, rushing pell-mell down the snack aisle, throwing things, most of them unhealthy, into the bottom of a shopping cart, and hoping there would be enough to feed everybody when he got back to the house. Which is to say, although it was obvious to him, it wasn't always clear to others what he was up to.

Because his was, after all, a university lab, Lynch was also a teacher, honored more than once as one of the best teachers at UCI. He was "the best prepared professor I've ever seen," another researcher recalled. "He'd spend two days prepping for a single lecture." Lynch was also one of UCI's most mischievous teachers. In lectures he frequently talked about the work being done in his lab, and he would heap praise on this or that fictitious grad student. He credited Garcia y Vega, the cigar manufacturer, with several important discoveries. He once described one of his star grad students, Kevin Lee, as "a little Chinese guy we keep in a closet." Lee, who is Scandinavian, would require a closet of some size; he is not a small man.

In other ways, Lynch was as unprofessorial as could be imagined. He had a wild head of hair, a scraggly beard, utterly mismatched teeth, and a chronic inability to refuse either a drink or a joint. If you were in the lab and weren't either hungover or about to be, you weren't really fitting in. What Lynch had, though, was manic energy, a wild charisma that drew people to the lab and kept them there no matter how many times he attacked a wall with a baseball bat.

Whatever one's expectations are of normal human behavior, finding these sorts of people did not prove to be all that difficult.

Typically, Lynch said, when he needed people, they seemed to just show up. Lee was a good example. He had come to the lab serendipitously. A native of suburban Los Angeles's San Gabriel Valley, he had attended the University of Southern California, which in the neuroscience world was not highly regarded. In 1974 he traveled to Irvine, about forty-five miles south of Los Angeles, for a summer school class, when a friend asked him to come play in a softball game. The friend said his lab needed a shortstop for the night. "The second baseman was this complete oddball, skinny guy," Lee recalled. "It was Gary. After the game, at the bar, Gary asked me who I was. I told him I was a recent psychology grad.

" 'Really,' he said. 'I thought you were just a ringer.' That's how I ended up in his lab.

"It was a wide-open world," Lee said. "We were all retread psychologists. This was exciting, and Gary was a master motivator. He instilled persistence. But if the lab wasn't as entertaining as it was, I'm not sure you'd make it through. It was a grand learning experience with Gary. He taught me that you need to decide what you need to do. Think of a problem you want to solve. Don't worry about how. We'll figure that out."

Lee arrived in mid-1974 at the same time as Mike Browning, an English major who had been hanging around Irvine after graduation working in a shoe store when he decided he wanted to become a neuroscientist. Neither Browning nor Lee was accepted into grad school on the first go-round. Browning, who habitually wore cut-off jeans, a cowboy hat, and boots, had even less formal training than Lynch in basic biology, but he intended to become a neuroscientist, whatever it took. He was required to pass a whole slate of basic undergraduate science classes before the grad school would even consider him for admission. He and Lee came to the lab anyway, joined the softball team, and worked there while they awaited admission.

The lab inhabitants as a rule were very bright, some of them brilliant. A number have gone on to chair university departments, to found successful companies, or to publish distinguished papers, but when they were in Lynch Lab, there wasn't much to recommend them to civil society. Any hint of future distinction was obscured by the sheer chain-gang grind.

In those early years—a period Lynch called "the boy lab" because of its testosterone-driven internal competitions—the lab was a woolly place, not far removed in its culture from a Neanderthal cave. Chris Gall, a grad student who would later become Lynch's significant other, was virtually the only woman. The guy with the biggest club generally got his way. Typically that was Lynch, who, though slight and not at all physically imposing, had a ferocious temper and never left a shadow of a doubt about his willingness to swing whatever was at hand. The place was littered with battered telephones and drywall with holes suspiciously the size of fists. "He never really hurt anybody physically but himself. Although there were people with emotional scars, I can tell you," said John Larson, a grad student in the lab's early days.

"That's part and parcel of the fire that burns in him," said Lee.

The phone on the wall? It just looked like a baseball sometimes. Chris was in the lab, but otherwise there were a lot of boys. I had a few issues myself. In that environment it seemed natural. You're bringing it pretty hard. There's a lot of competition. It's natural, something happens. Look at mice. Put enough of them in a cage for a while, they're ripping each other apart. There was a lot of macho in everything from science to beer drinking. Some people didn't make it, not because of the science, but because they couldn't do the whole not-sleeping thing.

"That lab was a strange, strange place to be at night, a lot of weird, weird, different kinds of people," Lynch recalled. "The dean would look at it and say, 'That's a strange damn place.'

"I'd answer: 'Have you looked at me?' "

Two notable properties of memory are its vast size and its time course—it can be made in moments, yet last for a lifetime. Any description of the physical components of memory has to account for those properties. There are roughly 100 billion neurons in the human brain. Each neuron has dozens of dendrites, and each dendrite can have thousands of synapses. The total number of synapses is estimated at anywhere from 100 trillion to many quadrillion. On whichever end of the scale the actual number falls, neuronal synapses clearly offer immense storage capacity, satisfying the first requirement for a storage mechanism.

But how could that storage be so long-lasting? "For me it was really, really obvious it had to be structural, but beyond that, what could I tell you?" Lynch said. "All along, going back to Princeton, I've been convinced that some level of information about structure will yield a lot of information about function, and any deep explanation has to start with neuroanatomy. I remember riding the train to Wilmington studying a rat neuroanatomy book. I was amazed at how much the circuitry explained."

His early LTP experiments persuaded Lynch that LTP was potentially a huge discovery. He decided to concentrate the lab's research on the search for the biological mechanism underlying memory. The course the initial investigations had to take was clear: the lab would become an LTP factory, seeking to determine what caused the potentiation effect and why it lasted. If LTP was the biochemical underpinning of memory, and if memory was encoded in networks of neurons, Lynch thought, something had to happen to the neuron itself during LTP. If the neuron weren't somehow made special, you could replace it with another. Clearly this didn't happen, so what did? From the beginning, from first principles, Lynch went looking for a physical change in neurons as the underlying basis of LTP.

"I came to it because it was the neatest problem in the world," Lynch said.

It was a mystery, and that's cool, a colossal mystery because there was no biological mechanism for it. Nothing. I loved LTP as a candidate for memory because the constraints on it from time zero, 1973, were so severe, there couldn't be that many answers. . . . There can't be many things that would do this in the biological universe. You come up asking how many known biological processes could match this little multidimensional hole: rapid appearance, stabilization in minutes, affects this synapse, but not one that's a micron away and possesses extraordinary persistence. These are independent dimensions, constraints. As Buffalo Bob used to say: "Jeez, that's gonna be a pretty tight fit, Howdy."

Lynch had a couple of exceptional postdocs, Sparky Deadwyler and Tom Dunwiddie, and a handful of promising graduate students, but to run the slice chamber experiments he needed an army. Lynch did few experiments himself. In part, this was due to an extreme allergy to rats, the main experimental animals used in the lab; beyond that, he simply didn't enjoy bench work much. Mainly he designed, assigned, or approved the experiments everyone else in the lab did. If a member of the lab was capable—sometimes even if he or she was not—Lynch would suggest a general idea and let the researcher conceive of a way to proceed. It was exhilarating for new grad students, for example, to be given the same long leash as the most experienced postdocs. They were also free to fail, and if they did so often, they weren't long for the lab—Lynch threw them out. In the end, he was a dictator, sometimes but not always benevolent.

Lee, not long after his arrival in 1974, was assigned the task of finding the physical change Lynch supposed LTP created. Lynch's extraordinary drive and rare ability to make every person feel that he or she was working on the single most important experiment in the history of neuroscience was the oxygen the lab lived on. He used his popularity and almost preposterous charm to recruit dozens of undergraduate students to work under Lee, running the slice chamber experiments day and night for months on end. "Memory was a great subject. And if it was going to be memory, then we thought it has to be something physical. I spent the next several years looking at synapses," Lee said. "It was a grind, as mindless as anything you'll ever do in your life."

The basic process, repeated a thousand times over, was this: A laboratory rat would be killed, its hippocampus removed from its brain and cut into very thin slices. The slices would be placed, one at a time, into the chambers the lab had developed; there they would be kept alive while electrodes were placed in them, one to stimulate an electrical current, another to measure the current as it passed through the slice.

After the stimulation, Lee's teams would apply a fixative to the slice to preserve it; they would stain it, cut it into still thinner slices, and mount these on thin polymer film. In a dimly lit room, they would view the slides and take photographs through an electron microscope, magnifying the images many thousands of times. The film would be developed and prints made. Like numbers of slides were made from the brains of a control group of animals, animals that had not been subjected to the electric stimulation. The two piles would be mixed together. Then Lee and the undergraduates would pore over the photographs, which looked, Lee said, "like mangled spaghetti with ink thrown on them," searching for abnormalities on the neurons in the images. "We did that blindly, just started looking for stuff," Lee said. "Changes in the spine structure, changes in the number of synapses. We were trying to determine the defining characteristic of the tissue absent knowing what we were looking at."

They circled with felt-tipped pens what seemed to be abnormalities on the images and sorted the photos into piles—those with and without the abnormalities. They did this for three years without any clear patterns emerging. The experiment lasted so long, it became the subject of a book-length academic study on the sociology of life in a laboratory. Lynch joked one day to his postdocs that he was going to move the whole lab into the animal colony, where the rats were raised, and not let anybody leave until either the rats were all dead or they had found the change he was looking for. It wasn't immediately clear he was kidding.

At times the search for the hypothesized physical change seemed ridiculous. How could you look that long for something and not find it? The most obvious answer was, the thing you were looking for didn't exist. It was the chance you took when you followed your intuition. The hope was—had to be—that the intuition was based on something more than desire. Lynch despaired but never wavered. "As far as I was concerned there was no other explanation," he said. "It got very ugly—holes in the walls, stuff tossed out of windows. But Kevin [Lee] was not going to back down. So if I wasn't going to stop, neither would he. It was like Guadalcanal."

Finally, one night in 1978, Lynch was routinely reviewing that day's stack of micrographs and their felt-tipped circles. In this particular stack of images, however, there were additional markings in the corners of some of the images. It wasn't obvious to Lynch what the additional markings were intended to indicate. He found the student, Mike Oliver, who had made the marks and asked what they meant. Oliver explained that though he hadn't found any of the four or five sorts of changes he had been trained to identify (mainly, enlarged dendritic spines), he had noticed the regular appearance of another anomaly. It seemed to be a different sort of synapse altogether, created along the shafts of some dendrites.

Lynch frantically tore through the stacks of the photographs, looking for similar changes. Sure enough, they were there. "I'll never forget," Lynch later said. "I was thinking, God, this can't be true, this can't be true. We've finally found something."

Changes had been occurring all along, just not the sort Lynch had anticipated. Later analysis estimated that the number of these synapses had increased by about a third in the experimental slices. Whether the synapses had been there all along, unseen, until increasing in size due to the experimental stimulation or were entirely new was unclear. Further investigation indicated that after the stimulation other spine heads changed shape, becoming more ovoid. The data were ambiguous but tantalizing. What was clear was that the same kind of stimulations that caused LTP also caused discernible changes in the physical structures of neurons at the synapses where they met. LTP changed the structure of the brain.

When the results were published two years later, nobody believed them. The basic reaction, Lynch said, was "How's a guy sitting out in Irvine able to discover stuff we haven't?" In many respects it didn't matter then to Lynch that no one believed the results. Very few people were routinely doing slice experiments—most of the field was still concentrated on a gene-based model for memory—so there was no conceivable way they could have duplicated the experiments. What mattered more to Lynch was that he was beginning to believe the results himself.

One of the uncomfortable realities of doing neurobiology is that you can almost never be certain what you are actually doing. Francis Crick, the codiscoverer of the structure of DNA, had in the latter portion of his career turned to the study of the brain, setting up shop eighty miles south of Irvine at the Salk Institute in La Jolla. Not long after he entered the field, he realized it was a fundamentally different sort of pursuit than anything to which he had been accustomed. He warned against using classical reductionist logic in the life sciences. Physics, Crick said, had

> powerful, deep and often counterintuitive general laws . . . What is found in biology is mechanisms, mechanisms built with chemical components and that are often modified by other, later mechanisms added to the earlier ones. While Occam's razor is a useful tool in the physical sciences, it can be a very dangerous implement in biology. It is thus very rash to use simplicity and elegance as a guide in biological research.

Biology, in other words, is a mess. In some ways, this prevents biologists from having the sort of confidence in their findings that is routine in other scientific endeavors. They are almost always in the dark and forced to proceed on some combination of hunch, estimation, and unwarranted conviction. "Don't feel bad if I don't believe your shit," Lynch said. "I don't believe my own shit."

With the successful conclusion of the micrograph work, Lynch was satisfied that LTP was a genuine phenomenon. Electrical stimulation of normal pathways in the hippocampus of mammals created a long-lasting increase in the flow of current through the pathways. That increased flow was accompanied by a physical change in the structure of neurons at the synapses (the places where they met other neurons). What did it mean? Was it anything more than a mere laboratory curiosity? These unresolved fundamental questions couldn't even be addressed until the phenomenon itself was far better understood.

One of Lynch's gifts as a scientist was his ability to frame questions in a clear and logical way, so that the answers, if found, would fit within the constraints of the system he was studying.

With LTP, he devised, and eventually the field adopted, a conceptual view that allowed him to lay out a clear research path. In his view LTP had three distinct stages—induction, expression, and consolidation. Put another way, there were three fundamental questions: How did the change occur? What was the actual change? Why did it last? The first question, now that the fact of a physical change had been demonstrated, was ready to be investigated.

The mood in the lab, after the long forced march and redeeming success of the micrograph experiment, was boisterous. One benefit of the years-long experiment was that in the process the scientists had perfected the slice methodology. They had designed and built their own equipment and protocols. So successful was the equipment design that, as knowledge of the slice technique spread, UCI's machine shop ran a cottage industry manufacturing slice chambers, and scientists came from all over the world to learn the technique. The flow of visitors through the lab was constant.

In the fall of 1978 Michel Baudry, an ambitious young biochemist from Paris, arrived in the lab, at the tail end of a five-week tour through the top U.S. neuroscience labs. He had funding from the French government for a postdoc in the United States and had already looked at labs at Harvard, Yale, in New York, and at the National Institutes of Health. "I came to Irvine at the end of my tour and met Gary. First, I was really surprised that Gary was so young. I had only seen all these publications he had [an astonishing eighty-four in the prior five years]. I thought, 'Shit, he's my age. And he's already done all this?' "

Baudry was even more surprised when, on the first evening of his Irvine visit, the entire lab emptied out at five p.m.; everybody left, including Lynch. "I said, 'Where are you all going?' They said they're going to a baseball game." It was softball actually, but Baudry was right in noting that the lab took its team seriously, or at least as seriously as one could when players took breaks between at-bats for a toke off a marijuana joint. There was also the somewhat disconcerting behavior of the shortstop, Lee, who sometimes provided play-by-play commentary as he was playing.

Amy Arai, a native of Japan who joined the lab soon after, recalled the culture shock she felt. "In Japan, everything is very formal. Scientists wear jackets and ties to work every day. Here in Irvine, nobody did that," she said.

> The whole thing was a big shock to me. All the big males. I had a hard time even locating Gary. He was never where he was supposed to be. I wandered around looking for him. There were lots of people wandering around, including one particularly scruffy guy I saw in the hallways, shirt always untucked and dirty. I'd sort of hold my breath when I passed him in the hall. I thought he was a janitor.

One day, weeks after she had arrived, Arai was summoned to Lynch's office, which by then was in a trailer next to a parking lot, far removed from the rest of the faculty offices. Arai walked in and found the trailer empty except for the janitor, who was sitting behind a desk smoking a cigar. It was Lynch. "He was very unconventional," she said. "He had no computer. He wrote everything on a yellow legal pad. Work was conducted through casual conversations. When he was interested in something, he'd stop by every day. Make a nuisance of himself, in fact."

The mixture of mad science and manic behavior that marked the Irvine lab was becoming legend throughout the neuroscience world. Neuroscience, like other academic disciplines, had established a regular rotation of conferences and seminars. Such annual and incidental meetings are fruitful places for the exchange of ideas and personnel, a cross-pollination that helps the science stay healthy and grow. They also tended to be fabulous parties. Lynch was becoming a roiling figure at these meetings, and not just because of his science. He is one of those people who, by accident or design, gathers a crowd almost wherever he goes.

At the annual Society for Neuroscience convention, a Lynch entrance was like an invasion, the Visigoths sweeping in off the distant plain, shredding the crops, stealing the women, sacking civil society. One Lynch colleague was so eternally ready for entertainment that he made a habit of sidling up to Lynch while he was engaged in conversation, and during the rare pauses he would ask, always, the same question: Is this going to help me get laid?

"He was a cult figure," said Alcino Silva of UCLA. "Or at least as close as we ever got in neuroscience. He was so charismatic."

It might have been as much generational as anything. The more respectable crowd, personified by Columbia University's Eric Kandel, with his continental background and Old World bow ties, were restrained and well mannered, at least in public. Lynch, meanwhile, was getting drunk at the bar and loudly proclaiming the silliness of all ideas that challenged his. Neuroscience in those years was a burgeoning enterprise, whose challenges drew eminent scientists of all backgrounds. "It was like battleship row," Lynch said. "All the ships lined up and ready to sail."

Lynch recalled giving a talk at one such meeting and being approached afterward by a man who congratulated him, then proceeded to ask a seemingly endless series of questions. The inquiries seemed insultingly commonplace to Lynch, who answered a few but indicated, without actually saying so, that, really, if you're interested in this stuff, you ought to get a bright grad student to explain it to you. When the man left, Lynch turned to one of his associates and said, in effect, Who was that idiot?

The friend said, You've heard of Cooper pairs?

Lynch assured his friend that he was well aware of the coupled electron pairing that was a key element of Leon Cooper's newly propounded theory of superconductivity. How could he not be? It was one of the great intellectual leaps of the century.

The friend said: That's Cooper.

Baudry, softball games notwithstanding, decided he couldn't afford to miss out on whatever was bound to happen next in Lynch's lab. He went back to Paris and informed his professors he was going to Irvine. When he told Jean-Pierre Changeux, the rising star of French neuroscience, that he was going to do a postdoc with Gary Lynch,

> he looked at me. He said, "You're crazy. Gary Lynch? The hippie of neurobiology?" Then I said the same thing to Henry Lester [another neuroscientist], who said, "Gary? He's going to be dead in three years. He does drugs, he smokes, he drinks." I said, "I'll take my chance." I went to Gary's lab, and it really was something different in its ambience. All these wild people. The contrast with Paris, fields, cows around the campus. I thought, I have to give this a shot. It really was the Wild West. And Gary really was this wild person.

Baudry arrived about the time Sam Deadwyler, a postdoc who had been a key collaborator with Lynch, left for a faculty position at Wake Forest. "Up until the day I left, I don't think Gary believed I was leaving," Deadwyler said. Indeed, it was Lynch who was often threatening to abscond. "Every other week he was going to take a job somewhere else. That was the joke— where's he going this week?"

Baudry initially was a bit overwhelmed. Tremendous excitement and commotion stirred in the lab. "People were coming from everywhere. My English was not very good. Even though I had taken it for fifteen years, I could not understand a word, and people could not understand a word I was saying," Baudry said. "There was a Polish postdoc in the lab, and we would speak English together, and we had no problem understanding each other. We'd talk, have long, vigorous conversations in English. Everybody around us understood nothing we were saying."

Baudry found the language-imposed isolation depressing. Additionally, he was having problems in his marriage; his wife returned to France. Coincidentally, Chris Gall, by then Lynch's girlfriend, finished her Ph.D. and went to the East Coast to do a postdoc. Baudry and Lynch were both suddenly single. "We spent a lot of time touring all the bars in Irvine," Baudry said. "We grew very close. Gary doesn't sleep. I got in the habit of not sleeping too. He's incredible. I don't know how he survives. I asked him once, 'What's your diet?' And Gary said: 'You don't want to know.' "

By every account, including his own, in those years Lynch ate badly, drank heavily, and slept hardly at all. On some days he seemed to consume more cigars than calories. His diet, in fact, was a subject of some fascination. For a long period, Lee said, the only things he ever saw Lynch eat came out of a vending machine, a single vending machine. His main meal, if you could call it that, consisted of salted peanuts mixed into soft drinks.

"You know, Gar," Lee told him, "you might think about diversifying your diet. Nothing radical, but hey, man, try a new machine. Have some chips."

Lynch's diet was of a piece with his extreme work habits, which typically included seven days a week of twelve-hour or longer stints in the lab, often followed by monumental bouts in the nearest bar. On nights when, for whatever reason, they couldn't get to the bar, Lynch held long, rambling, off-the-cuff seminars in his office. They were open to all comers—students, postdocs, collaborators, junior faculty; if you could scrounge up a six-pack of beer as the price of admission, you were welcome to attend. Lynch presided, Budweiser in one hand, piece of chalk in the other, diagramming the pathways of the hippocampus one moment, analyzing elliptical Neil Young lyrics the next, and squeezing in comparisons of Einstein to horror movies in between. He saw it all as essential to the education of young scientists.

"He always tells us he isn't interested in nurturing electrophysiologists or biochemists," said Amy Arai. "He nurtures neuroscientists. One of my advantages is I have a very good enzyme in my liver. I can drink a lot of beer."

The sessions provided an outlet as well as a training ground for lab members who had questions or complaints, which they did—about pay, about whose names went on which papers, about whose turn it was to buy booze.

"It was so competitive in the lab, nobody would tell you when something was wrong. You had to figure it all out. Nobody would tell you anything," said Ursula Stäubli, a Swiss postdoc who came during this period. "Once you're in Gary's lab, he makes you work so hard. You get home at ten o'clock, eat some chips for dinner, fall asleep. My whole life became work. It was exciting, and he kind of makes it that way. After a while, you know, 'This is going to make you famous,' or 'That is going to.' You believe that for maybe a year. It was always very exciting."

"I was pretty competitive. So was everybody else. You got what you grabbed," said John Larson, a quiet but intense midwesterner who had come to the lab at the suggestion of one of Lynch's competitors, William Greenough of the University of Illinois.

In the midst of all that was happening in the lab, Lynch, still just a very young professor, was unexpectedly asked to serve as his academic department's chairman. The psychobiology department was aptly named, he said, if for no other reason than that they asked him to run it. "The dean came to me one day and said, 'You know, Lynch, I don't much like you, but I think you ought to be the chairman.'"

It's worth noting that at this point, 1983, Lynch still looked (and sometimes acted) more like Charles Manson than a university department head. He asked the dean two questions.

I said, "(A) Why would you possibly want me to be the chairman?" He was offended by me, by my lifestyle.

He said: "This is a really good department. It has a chance to be the best department in the world. And as much as I hate to admit it, apparently you're really good at this shit. So you should be chairman."

I went, "Well, that explains A, but (B) Why should I do it?"

He put it on me: "You owe it."

I said, "Okay."

You've never seen a shock like this: "Gary's the chairman. Oh. My. God."

He did the job for three years, all the while running the lab at full speed and his life on the outer edges of sanity. Typically for insurgents who end up taking command, he insisted things get done in a way that he himself would have rebelled against. He made researchers teach and gave students an opportunity to learn. "It's easy to build a great department," he said. "You just have to put up with assholes.

In terms of biological sciences, we were as good as you could get and it wasn't that hard to do it. I used to give a speech to the introductory biology students: "Here's the thing. You kids understand something. What you get here is maybe not everything you would have at some other place, but if you work with us, there will be no better education on this fucking planet. So you little sonsabitches understand that. If you work here, there will be no better education on this planet. We have the faculty here that will take you into their laboratories, they will let you be performing at the level of a postdoctoral fellow within three weeks. You have chances here you will have no other place. Nobody will be better."

CHAPTER FOUR

A New and Specific Hypothesis

CALPAIN, EARLY 1980S

If the LTP hypothesis were true, then the constituent elements of the process demanded understanding. As usual, Lynch knew nothing about the basic subject—cell biology—he was proposing to invade. He nonetheless decided there had to be a biochemical remodeling of cell interiors in order to produce the structural change they had found under Lee's microscope. Lynch knew that cell shape was not random but was generally determined by an assemblage of internal proteins that formed an interior cytoskeleton.

Even before Lee's experiment confirmed the shape-change, Lynch was convinced it existed and had started burrowing through the existing cell biology literature. He thought it would be nice if he didn't need to invent new biology but could borrow some that already existed. It's a lot less work, he said. He had concluded that one of the first steps in the LTP process was driven by calcium, which exists in large but uneven quantities in the brain in the extracellular space, the areas between neurons. He had published a paper proposing that LTP was more likely to occur and be stronger in areas where the extracellular calcium existed in higher concentrations. That gave him a hint of where in the cell biology literature to search. "I was looking for small cells that underwent rapid, calcium-dependent shape-changes," he said.

Sudden shape-changes scared me, so I went looking for an instance in which cells could do this in a couple of minutes,

and came across platelets. And found it was calcium dependent. And then looked for calcium-dependent enzymes that
could help reorganize the platelet cytoskeleton. I needed an
enzyme that was going to be activated by calcium that was
going to change the cytoskeletal structure, relax it.

The word *reorganize* is something of a euphemism here.
These particular types of enzymes, called proteases, don't reorganize anything—they cut things apart. More to the point, they
cut specific things apart. What Lynch wanted was to find a protease whose assigned task was to cut up neural cell cytoskeletons.
"One happy day" in 1979, while browsing through abstracts in
the *Journal of Biological Chemistry,* he found a paper describing
an enzyme that disassembled the cytoskeletons of blood platelets
as part of the process by which platelets change shape and form
clots. The enzyme was called calpain. Typically in biology, molecules that do one thing in one place do some version of that same
thing in other places. Collagen, for example, one of the most
ubiquitous structural proteins, is present in everything from
bones to muscles to blood vessels. In each case it adds strength to
the structure. Calpain had not previously been identified as an
active neural enzyme, but scientists had long before developed
methods to determine whether particular molecules exist in specific tissues. It was a tedious but more or less routine matter for
Lynch to confirm that calpain, in fact, exists in the mammalian
brain. When he did so, he thought he had identified two big
pieces of the LTP-process puzzle—the calcium trigger and calpain, the thing the calcium activates.

Meanwhile, two different research groups—one in Denmark
and one in Canada—had found two other pieces. Both were
types of molecules called receptors. Neurons are not physically
connected to one another; a tiny space called a synaptic cleft
exists between the axon of one and the dendrite of another.
When neurotransmitters are released from the axon of one neu-

ron, they drift across the cleft. On the surface of the neighboring neurons are molecules that receive the neurotransmitters. These are the receptors. Think of the neurotransmitters as keys and the receptors as locks. When a neurotransmitter attaches to a receptor on the surface of a receiving cell—when the key opens the lock—channels open through the cell membrane into the interior of the cell. Because neurons are not connected, communication between them is never certain—you never know if a key is going to find a lock. In fact, there is only about a one-in-three chance that the neurotransmitter will even be released. This is one reason why any cognitive activity, including memory, is at best approximate. Sometimes the connections are made; other times they are not.

The first of these receptor discoveries was made in 1982 by Terje Honoré in Denmark. He found that on the receiving-cell side of the synapse, called the postsynaptic side, there is a receptor that when activated by the neurotransmitter glutamate opens a channel that allows sodium into the postsynaptic cell. This receptor would later be named the AMPA receptor (short for alpha-amino-3-hydroxy-5-methyl-4-isoxazole propionic acid; oddly, most receptors are named not for their own characteristics but for the chemical structures of other molecules that bind to them). A year later Graham Collingridge, a British postdoc working in a Canadian lab, discovered that glutamate also locks onto a second receptor known as the NMDA receptor (N-methyl D-aspartate).

It turned out that the NMDA receptor opens only when it receives glutamate after the AMPA receptor has already been opened. Together they constitute a dual switch that relies on precise timing. There have to be two spikes in the axon, the first spike priming the postsynaptic cell through the AMPA receptor, the second opening the cell to the flow of calcium through the NMDA receptor. In Irvine, Lynch greeted the receptor discoveries with open arms but also regret: he was irritated particularly that Collingridge had beaten him to the NMDA receptor. "Carl Cotman and I were on it, but he and I were having a primate bumping contest," Lynch said, and the time wasted resolving their alpha-male priorities cost them the discovery. Nonetheless, the fact that NMDA allows the calcium influx encouraged Lynch.·

Calpain became the central focus of the lab for several years. "They had slices going every day from dawn to midnight," said John Larson. Even at that rate it took years to gather enough evidence to publish the first calpain papers, which in neuroscience was not unusual. After Sam Deadwyler left for Wake Forest, Michel Baudry assumed Deadwyler's role as Lynch's chief collaborator. Deadwyler had been in the lab almost as long as Lynch and was widely respected and liked. Some of the other researchers saw Baudry as an interloper and resented him. But there was no doubting the results.

In 1984 Lynch and Baudry published an extraordinary paper in *Science.* "The Biochemistry of Memory: A New and Specific Hypothesis" summarized Lynch Lab's decade of work on LTP and postulated what it all meant. It made a strong argument for calpain's central role in dismantling the cell skeleton, then proposed (based on what Lynch termed "crappy evidence") how that skeleton might be rebuilt. The paper was audacious on several counts. The hypothesis was a direct challenge to the neuroscience establishment, which had continued to preach that memory was the result of some sort of unfound and unspecified protein synthesis. The fact that the protein-synthesis crowd, led by Eric Kandel, had yet to find anything but the most general support for their thesis made the Lynch–Baudry promise of a "specific" hypothesis almost a taunt.

The paper also entirely ignored the cultural convention that had evolved within the field to not talk much about LTP as a potential memory mechanism. You could think it, but it was considered gauche to say it. Lynch bluntly stated the largest ambitions possible, starting with the title and moving on from there. The paper laid out a course of research that would occupy him for at least the next two decades.

"Nobody in their right mind would ever imagine that you would turn this enzyme on and things would never be the same again," Lynch said, speaking of calpain.

It's a protease, and it eats the cytoskeleton, so you do not want it. You want it turned on briefly and discreetly because you know things will never be the same. Because you have just kicked the shit out of the cytoskeleton. As far as I was concerned, that was why the hypothesis had to be right. This process here is inherently dangerous. You let the calcium come in, you activate the deadly calpain. . . . It's a shark.

One time, Eric [Kandel] and I were someplace, and he's talking about kinases, and I'm talking about calpain. Blah, blah, blah. So I say, "Let's take your enzyme and my enzyme and put them in a test tube together and see who comes out. Then we'll know." Calpain—give it enough time, it'll eat anything. It would. You put anything in there, any protein in there for half an hour, it'll start eating it. Bad stuff.

Almost no one agreed with Lynch and Baudry that calpain played a fundamental role in LTP. One reason was precisely that everyone understood that calpain had such a destructive capacity. Lynch recognized it, but what others saw as a problem, he saw as proof. A fundamental difficulty in hypothesizing a memory mechanism is the nature of the brain itself. Most cells in the body turn over with some regularity, in some parts every few days or weeks. Most biological change derives to some extent from this cellular replacement. But the hundreds of billions of neural cells in the brain, once they mature, stay for as long as the brain lasts. And new cells are not routinely added. In fact, many more neurons die during a lifetime than are added. With some exceptions, the population of neurons you start out with is the population of neurons you go to the grave with. Memory, by definition, is the retention of newly acquired information. If new information does not come in new cells, the old ones have to change, and they have to change fast given the rate at which brains can acquire information.

Calpain can initiate almost instant change inside a neuron's dendrites. Yes, it was true, Lynch agreed, calpain could be dangerous, and many of the malfunctions of the brain as it aged might well be due to calpain's destructive appetites. That sort of trade-off is a common outcome of random evolutionary change. Memory is good, but in order to get it, you have to accept the possibility of occasional disaster.

"When you built this great learning mechanism, you did two things that were bound to be fatal in the end," Lynch said.

One is you fixed it so that these branches [the dendrites] are incredibly stable; they don't turn over, otherwise you lose the memory. Secondly, to knock out that stability with a protease using a very complicated, sharp fashion, that same protease, calpain, has no known function other than feeding. This was an enzyme in search of something to do. This, of course, was my point. The double deal you made with the devil: you go to stability, and the technology you're using to dismantle stability, it goes a little too far, you're done. I think that's what goes on in the brain with aging.

In the late 1980s, Lynch preached the calpain hypothesis to anyone who would listen, and to many who would not. It gained almost no traction.

It finally dawned on me that nobody cared about calpain. I don't think they understood the problem. I think in large measure because nobody understood that if you change the shape of the dendritic spine, you change the function of the synapse. Calpain wasn't hypothesized. I didn't give a hoot in hell about calpain. I didn't know anything about calpain at all. I just needed something to destabilize the spine. I really thought this is going to excite people, because look at how exotic this is—a calcium-driven protease, ya know? Nobody, hardly anybody in the world noticed. Some Japanese group came out, who were really cool calpain guys, and said it doesn't even exist in the brain. This was after I published a paper saying it was the cause of LTP.

Lynch stopped for a moment, pointed his index finger, pistol style, at his head, and pulled the trigger three times. "Bang. Bang. Bang. No calpain in the brain, huh? I was amazed. Nobody sees how extraordinary this enzyme is. I deal with these guys, then some guy on the East Coast is going, 'There's no spectrin in the brain, no structural protein in the brain, you can't be measuring it.' "

Lynch screwed up his face like a rodeo clown getting ready to humiliate a bull. "What the fuck do you think we're measuring?"

Lynch, in moments like this, virtually jumps out of his chair. Not screaming, exactly, but very nearly squealing. Then he settled back, resigned. "It's unbelievable," he said. "You feel like Frederick the Great in the Seven Years' War: Marie's over here, the Russians over here, the French are over there. You can't get a moment's breath."

Baudry was somewhat more prosaic: "We had the feeling we were making important new discoveries, that we were on the frontier. It was perplexing."

MAGIC RHYTHM, LATE 1980S

Nobody discounted Lynch's brilliance. Indeed, he became for a time a nearly famous person. *The New York Times* featured the calpain hypothesis in its Sunday magazine, which put Lynch on the media map as a go-to guy for comment on almost anything. The *Times* attended to him. The BBC came calling for a documentary on memory. Dutch television wanted his thoughts on what constituted true beauty. Lynch, of course, had answers for everyone. Often the answers were thoughtful, more informed than anyone had a right to expect. Neuroscience is filled with very smart people, but even among them Lynch stood out. One former member of his lab said that Lynch is one of those rare people who, within five minutes of meeting him, you know you are in the presence of an intellectual giant. But a notion was emerging in the field that maybe Lynch was too smart for his own good, that he was so good at devising clever explanations that he didn't take the time to gather evidence to support them. Lynch thought just the opposite—that he was out there doing the scut work of true science, charging headfirst into every wall in sight to gather every shred of evidence he could. His competitors, he thought, were too busy chasing magic genes and silver-bullet proteins to join him down in the biochemical muck where the real answers lay.

The calpain disagreement was in fact the first round of a debate that would polarize the field for the next fifteen years. The issue was: did the fundamental activity that caused LTP to persist happen on the axon side of the synapse (the so-called presynaptic side) or on the dendritic spine (the postsynaptic side)?

This polite intellectual disagreement would devolve into a feud, one that lacked none of the ignorance, pigheadedness, and prejudice of any other feud. Scientists didn't take up arms, Hatfield-McCoy style, but in this fight, for a very long time, they acted every bit as stupidly as moonshine-crazed hillbillies.

The depth of the disagreement was probably more fundamental than either side cared to admit. Much of the neuroscience establishment simply did not accept LTP as anything

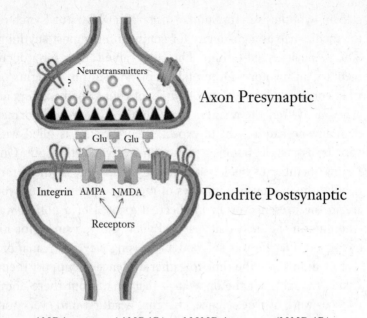

AMPA receptors (AMPAR) and NMDA receptors (NMDAR) both sit in the cell membrane on the postsynaptic side of the synapse. Glutamate (Glu) is released from the presynaptic side and drifts across the synaptic cleft. LTP occurs only when glutamate opens first the AMPA receptor, then the NMDA receptor. (Courtesy of Lynch Lab)

more than a laboratory phenomenon. They didn't think it had much if anything to do with memory. Even Lynch, to some extent, doubted the reality of what he was doing. "It was fun," he said. "Then you get to the thing, this is real, this is memory. A week later you start having these profound problems. Intellectually, what would it mean? Jesus Crikey. You believe it. Then the doubts come. They start pouring in. It's a new worry, a whole new set of worries. It's a big fucking deal."

In many respects, the LTP skeptics had a good argument. LTP was created by applying electrical stimulation to previously identified circuits in the hippocampus. How much current? For how long? How often? The experimental paradigms being employed for LTP experiments were, to put it kindly, diverse. Ideally researchers, in order to make experimental conditions as natural as possible, would model their experiments on rhythms known to occur within mammalian biology. Or, at least, as much as you could when your model for the brain was a slice of tissue the size of a nail clipping, long removed from its former owner and submerged in a tiny plastic swimming pool of oxygenated warm water. Lynch's initial incredulity regarding brain-slice efficacy had long since disappeared, and he championed the technique, but especially in LTP's early years a healthy suspicion of it remained in the field.

Somehow the combination of the slice technique and the artificial stimulation lent the whole affair a dubious quality. The big variable was the electrical stimulation. Perhaps in part because of the distrust of the technique itself, some labs did little to honor natural conditions, applying levels of stimulation far beyond what anyone could defend as natural. Lynch was critical of the wanton lack of experimental consistency across the field. "Give me control of that [electric] knob, and I can make anything happen," he said. On the other hand, knowledge of the natural rhythms of the brain was insufficient.

John Larson, who had come from Chicago to Lynch Lab as a grad student just as the calpain hypothesis was developed, began a series of experiments in 1986 to determine the optimal stimulation pattern to obtain LTP. The stimulation had three variables: the intensity of the electric current, the pattern of it (that is, how often it would be applied), and the duration of the application. This was, in many ways, a typical grad student project. Somebody else in the lab was doing something that involved using lizard tails for an experiment. "So," Larson said, "we had a lot of lizard brains going to waste." Larson put them to use. He began a systematic exploration of how different stimulations affect LTP. "Most people were using long trains, more than a second of stimulation. Gary favored ultrahigh frequencies. It turned out it didn't work any better than other frequencies. What floored us was that the assumption had always been that more stimulation is better. It wasn't. If you threw out most of it, it worked better."

The optimal stimulation turned out to be near the middle of the range. LTP was strongest when the time between bursts was about 200 milliseconds, equal to the rate of approximately five per second, or five hertz. This rate was remarkably similar to a natural rhythm in the mammalian brain, called theta rhythm, that had been discovered in the mid-1950s and occurs in the hippocampus when an animal is alert and exploring new environments. It is, in other words, the brain rhythm that occurs during learning. "Everybody always wondered what it was there for," Larson said.

Larson's discovery fit perfectly with the earlier reports of the two-step receptor switches for opening channels into the receiving neuron. The spacing of the stimulation bursts in the theta rhythm exactly matched the spacing required to first prime the NMDA receptor, then open it. If there was no space between bursts, the NMDA receptor didn't open. If there was too much time between bursts, it didn't open. Theta gave the lab an understanding of the NMDA receptor that would have been impossible without it.

The linkage between theta rhythms and NMDA receptor activation goes back to lamprey eels. That a rhythm originating with locomotion through water would eventually evolve into a rhythm associated with human learning is an example of the peculiarities of evolution, and of the truism that evolution doesn't care what tools it has, only how to use them.

"That day—the day we found theta—our mouths fell open. The shock isn't that it worked, but that it was the best possible rhythm. People were using lots of stimulations. Now we knew that stimulation conditions were well within what happens in real life," Lynch said, adding that the correspondence of theta with the dual receptors was "excruciatingly elegant." This coincidence—that the best way to obtain LTP in the lab was to mimic actual real-world biology—more than anything that had come before persuaded Lynch that LTP could be real. "When theta stimulation turned out to be the same as the natural rhythms, that was too much of a coincidence," he said. "I mean, God's a prick, but come on. He can't be that mean.

> I realized, and so did Larson, that we had uncovered some kind of basic rule for association. Back there in Princeton I had taken a course on the history of psychology with a wild man named Julian Jaynes [who] introduced me to associationism, Bishop Berkeley, Hume, and, much as I hate to admit it, I loved that shit. So yeah, when we got the theta thing, I immediately thought of the law of contiguity. Larson and I went on to carry out experiments which pushed the issue. We started to think about how time determines whether or not disparate elements, letters, are recognized as a single word or two words. Nobody gave a fuck . . . but I will always regret not following up on that paper. It was the beginning of a set of rules for how time—contiguity—inevitably shapes what is called the same, or called different. A year of research and you'd have rules of surprising richness, empirically grounded rules for why information must be assembled in the way it is. Manny Kant stuff, [Noam] Chomsky stuff, all just laying there.

The discovery of theta, although it wasn't widely recognized at the time, moved LTP from the it-could-not-possibly-be-true category of laboratory artifact to the more mundane classification of just-another-brain-state. It had long been recognized that the brain operates at different times at different rhythms. The rhythms are the result of neurons firing their electrical signals, called action potentials. Neurons fire these action potentials, or spikes, at various rates depending on what the brain is doing. Action potentials are a nearly constant process in an awake brain, firing at a rate of up to seventy times per second, the so-called gamma rhythm. If the rhythm is slowed down to five spikes per second, the memory machine kicks in. This makes intuitive sense. The world buzzing by at seventy times a second is little more than a blur. Slowing it down made keeping track of what went on possible, gave the memory machinery time to work. LTP, if theta was indeed its natural rhythm, was nothing more than the adaption of the action potential to a novel use—record keeping.

Lynch thought the discovery of theta closed out the investigation of the first phase of LTP—induction. Theta rhythms caused axons to fire in a pattern that opened first the AMPA receptor, then the NMDA receptor, allowing extracellular calcium to pour into the receiving neuron. The calcium activated the calpain protease, kicking off the next stage of the process—called, in Lynch's schematic view, expression.

At its essence, LTP is the phenomenon of a persistent increase in the amount of current passed between two cells. If he was to ever persuade his critics, or even himself, that the calpain hypothesis was correct, Lynch had to work out the details of the multistep process that causes the increased current. He felt he knew what LTP was and when it occurred. Now he had to work out the details of what actually happened. He spent much of the next decade on the problem.

One way an individual receptor could allow more current to pass would be to reduce the electrical resistance in the receptor channel through which the current travels. Lynch already had evidence that the spine head changes to a slightly rounder shape. In principle, this would reduce internal resistance. It was the simplest if not necessarily the likeliest hypothesis. Largely using pharmacological manipulations, the lab tried over a couple of years to demonstrate this reduction but never was able to do so.

Eventually Lynch gave up on the idea. Ruling out the resistance argument left him three other possibilities:

- The presynaptic neuron could release more of the neurotransmitter, presumed to be glutamate, from its axon.
- Each receptor could stay open longer, increasing the amount of calcium entering the postsynaptic cell and eventually the amount of current.
- The postsynaptic neuron could add receptors, which would have the same effect as the original receptors staying open longer.

The first possibility—the release of more neurotransmitter—seemed unlikely, because the axon terminal didn't appear to have the machinery inside it to be modulated. "The terminals are primitive, crude things, just big bags of water," Lynch said. The neurotransmitters were contained inside small vesicles inside the terminals, and release of them upon an electrical spike was biologically a pretty simple event. It was fundamental and ingenious, effectively converting an electrical signal into a chemical signal, but very straightforward. Plus, almost everyone in the field now agreed that LTP induction occurred on the postsynaptic side, along the lines Lynch had laid out. How would the presynaptic side—the axon terminal—even know to release more neurotransmitter? It would presumably require some sort of retrograde signal back across the synapse, but no such signal or signaling mechanism was known to exist. The synapse, as Cajal had first hypothesized and so far as anyone could tell, was a one-way street.

The improbability of the presynaptic argument did not stop respected scientists from advancing it. Chief among them was Eric Kandel, the most prominent and powerful figure in all of neuroscience. Kandel headed the Howard Hughes Medical Institute's Center for Neurobiology and Behavior at Columbia Uni-

versity, in almost every respect at the opposite end of the neuroscience universe from Lynch Lab, at a state school in the suburban sprawl of southern California. Lynch's office was a trailer in a
parking lot. Kandel's office, in a midrise tower, commanded a
sweeping view of the Hudson River. Lynch's university lacked
tradition and was strikingly middlebrow. The Hughes Institute
was the richest private funder of science in the United States.
Lynch's lab was filled with hippies and castoffs. Kandel's lab was
filled with an army of disciplined, career-tracked strivers. Lynch
was a wild man, Kandel the model of discretion. Lynch made
every pronouncement imaginable in the public square; Kandel
was a master backroom politician.

Kandel had become a kind of godfather of contemporary
neuroscience, widely acknowledged—and in many places reviled. He was regarded with both awe and loathing. Scientists
blamed him for losing grants, faculty positions, and even funding for biotech start-ups. Some became so agitated in talking
about him, they would sputter and scream. Once, when I was
interviewing a prominent researcher, I mentioned Kandel in
passing, and within two minutes the man, whom I had just met,
was shouting invective, at one point while standing atop his desk.

Competitors sometimes rolled their eyes when asked what
Kandel's standing derived from. They were somewhat disingen-
uous about it. Beyond any single discovery, Kandel's investigations into synaptic plasticity had pushed and shaped the field as
it was being born. That he continued to wield great influence, if
not actual power, was evidenced by the prominence that the
study of protein synthesis enjoyed within memory research.
Lynch thought the emphasis was wrongheaded, but he could do
little to overcome it. Kandel, for his part, had nothing but nice
things to say about Lynch.

If it seemed inevitable that Kandel and Lynch would disagree, in some ways they were alike. Both men were widely read

outside their fields and essentially self-educated within it. As undergraduates, Lynch had majored in psychology, Kandel in history. "We're both dilettantes," Lynch said.

Kandel, who was a generation older than Lynch, had been a pioneer in moving the study of the mind from an investigation of behavior to an investigation of molecules. He had made his greatest discoveries by spending decades working out the bio-chemical mechanisms that underlay learning behaviors in a very primitive animal—*Aplysia californica*, the simple sea slug. Kandel proposed that *Aplysia* could be used as a model system for studying learning and memory generally. He discovered the neural underpinnings of the slug's most basic learned responses, demonstrating for the first time that molecular mechanisms were indisputably the basis of at least some forms of learning. In a sense, he legitimized the field of neurobiology. Kandel's desire to anchor vague concepts of learning and memory in molecular behavior was exactly the same motivation that drove Lynch to abandon psychology. Kandel was convinced that the fundamen-tal changes that LTP precipitated in the mammalian brain oc-curred presynaptically, as they did in *Aplysia*. This belief was shared by, among others, Tim Bliss, who had returned to the field with a series of papers in which he claimed to have mea-sured an increase in glutamate dispersion from the presynaptic axon terminals during LTP.

Lynch couldn't for the life of him figure out why anyone would think this was so. He thought that memory mechanisms, whatever they turned out to be, were relatively recent evolution-ary inventions, appearing long past the evolution of Kandel's sea slug. What was the practicality of studying memory in nonmam-mals that, in human terms, didn't have any? Lynch wondered. He joked about it: "Eric, come on, we haven't had a common ancestor for five hundred fifty million years. You don't think things could have changed?" More seriously, he said: "Memory is an emergent phenomenon. Steam is an emergent phenomenon. If you want to study steam, you better study hot water. You ain't going to get steam out of mud."

Lynch Lab examined Bliss's results. Marcus Kessler, a Swiss neurochemist, did most of the work. Kessler, in addition to being the de facto everyday manager of the lab, was a precise, fastidiously careful scientist, so careful, in fact, that he often riled other members of the lab, including Lynch, by questioning their work. Apparently alone among members of the lab, he seemed utterly resistant to Lynch's charms. In fact, he had been preparing to leave the lab to return to Switzerland before he fell in love with a newly arrived biologist, Amy Arai. He stayed for her, not for Lynch.

Bliss reported that he had been able to actually measure the increase in glutamate release. Kessler replicated the experiments Bliss described but found no such evidence. "Kessler has this really great formal training in science, which I certainly don't have. I don't have any training in science," Lynch said. "Kessler looked at Tim's results and was just, 'Ooooooh, I cannot believe someone was publishing this, because it is not possible.' "

Lynch Lab—with another Swiss postdoc, Dominique Muller, taking the lead—began doing experiments using a variety of pharmacological manipulations, blocking first one type of receptor, then the other, to measure under what circumstance the current increased. What they found was that passing more calcium—presumably the effect that adding more glutamate would have—through the NMDA receptor did not increase potentiation. Opening the NMDA door was a necessary but not sufficient condition for LTP. The AMPA receptor was absolutely determinant. You had to have both. Imagine the receptors as a set of double doors: nothing would fit through unless both doors were opened. It seemed definitive proof that the variables that controlled LTP were located in the postsynaptic cell.

In 1988 Roger Nicoll, at the University of California, San

Francisco, published virtually the identical conclusion simultaneously with Lynch. (That rankled Lynch more than he would admit. He couldn't figure out how Nicoll had been able to rush his paper from revision to publication in six weeks, while Lynch's waited the maddeningly normal many months. It would thereafter be a shared discovery—Nicoll 1988, Lynch 1988—in every citation made.) That both Nicoll and Lynch independently arrived at nearly identical results made a strong case that they were right, and Lynch chalked it up as another victory for his broader hypothesis.

"Game, set, match. That's kind of the dividing point in the history of LTP, that paper," he said. "When this thing came out, then everybody started going, It's postsynaptic, it's glutamate receptors. More glutamate receptors or changed glutamate receptors. And it's so much more economical to say more. The basic mechanism I described in that '84 *Science* paper ['The Biochemistry of Memory'] was, you change the shape of the spine, it's got more space for receptors, so you've got more receptors."

The presynapticists didn't give up. From the outside, many aspects of this debate seemed inconsequential. Who really cared at which side of the synapse this or that chemical reaction occurred? But much more was at stake here than pushing the science ahead an inch or so in one direction or the other. Bruce McNaughton, a presynapticist from the University of Arizona, put it succinctly years later: "People saw Stockholm at the end of the road." McNaughton was exactly right. There were few biological heights to scale as obvious and as towering as learning and memory. Gambling that LTP was the underpinning of memory might have been a long shot, but it was a bet with obvious payoffs. The one who won the bet would be standing on very high ground indeed, and wearing a Nobel medal.

The presynapticists proposed several different candidates as their hypothetical "second messenger," the molecule that would, after LTP was induced, travel back across the synapse to the presynaptic side and somehow cause an increase in glutamate release. They lacked mechanisms by which their candidates would trigger new release; they even failed for a long time to find some of the candidate compounds anywhere near the synapse. The whole notion of a second messenger remained purely theoretical, and because of that their argument flagged. Scientists, however, are extremely reluctant to give up a position they have previously published. Admissions of defeat are almost unheard-of. So they kept on.

In 1990 Richard Tsien and Charles Stevens, highly regarded electrophysiologists working in competing labs at Yale, resurrected the presynaptic argument. In simultaneously published but separate papers they claimed to have used a new method called quantal analysis to measure the release of neurotransmitter vesicle by vesicle (an astonishing claim, if true) and to have found that the release from the presynaptic side increased after LTP was induced, helping to maintain it.

"This changes the entire neuroscience world. This is the earthquake we've all been waiting for. Blah, blah, blah," Lynch said. "This is when my friend Larry Squire [from the University of California, San Diego] came up to me and said, 'Man, they just killed you. You're done. You're not talking about little boys here—this is Sir Charles and Dirty Dick. They got ya.' "

As it turned out, they didn't have him at all. The basic assumptions for the Tsien-Stevens manipulations were logically flawed. So obvious was the flaw that Tim Tully, a prominent LTP researcher then at Cold Spring Harbor, said a grad student of his figured it out within a day of reading the papers. The same thing happened at Lynch Lab—a student pointed out questionable assumptions Tsien and Stevens had made.

"Nonetheless," Tully said, "for four years, that's all you could hear: quantal analysis. None of that literature exists now. It's not polite or courteous to mention it."

CHAPTER FIVE

Exile

The direction of science is largely determined by the tools available to pursue it. Once, those tools amounted to little more than a clear eye and an analytical inclination. Over the centuries, and especially in the last hundred years, new technologies have supplanted old technologies with gathering speed, sophistication, and expense. Some contemporary sciences—high energy physics, astronomy, and genomics, to name a few—can hardly be approached now without access to a treasury the size of a small nation's.

Although these new technologies have made discoveries possible—indeed, they've revealed vistas hardly even imagined beforehand—they have not always led research in the most fruitful directions. The direction of science is not necessarily the same thing as the progress of science. Problems can arise when tools dictate direction, an illustration of the axiom that if you have only a hammer, every problem looks like a nail. Grant-makers and journal editors demand that you use the popular tools to gain their approvals. Tenure committees make decisions based on grants and publications. In very short order, basic research, which is supposed to be innovative, even radical, becomes staid and normative. Every neuroscientist has received a review asking him why he didn't use such-and-such technique, whether or not relevant, to do such-and such experiment. Interlopers are shunned, and risk-taking is constrained.

"The answer is being driven by the method du jour," Lynch

said. "If you've got a method that lets you look at something, then the answer must be what that method allows you to see. That is really what drives the field, that blinds them. It's probably a human condition. Science is refined, but is still an exercise in a certain human style."

In the early 1990s Lynch made an obligatory effort to refute the new quantal analysis claims being put forth by the presynaptic campaigners, but he grew dispirited about the whole business. It became personal in some respects. A sort of bandwagon effect developed. People who had been waiting for Lynch to get his comeuppance rejoiced. When scientists from Lynch Lab gave talks at various meetings, they were vigorously attacked for not taking the quantal analysis into consideration. The presynapticists seemed to Lynch to be indulging in wishful thinking. "They're electrophysiologists. They can't do anatomy. They can't do chemistry. All they can do is electrodes; therefore the answer must be at the end of an electrode. This is where I was an idiot. I just didn't take it seriously. I never took their quantal analysis seriously."

That others did depressed Lynch. It reinforced his notion that neurobiology wasn't a real science; it's not, he said, "a fit thing for a grown man to do." People said the damnedest things, things that couldn't possibly be true. And they were taken seriously. Where were the constraints? Where was the science?

"You cannot do that [say untrue things] in the physical sciences," Lynch said. "Well, you can, but it's called cold fusion. In neuroscience it's called a string of papers in *Nature.* You can impose your desires and your suspicions. That is the secret of biology. There's nothing that keeps you from saying that. You don't have those restraints."

Lynch liked to cite a common type of experiment, called fear learning, that had been used regularly over a period of decades and seemed to him to illustrate an utterly unhinged aspect of his field. In these experiments, rats or other animals were placed in cages, the floors of which were electrified grids. The rats would walk onto a portion of the floor and get shocked by the current; then they were removed and brought back sometime later. Predictably, the rats were skittish about getting shocked again. This would then be promoted as an example of learning. Once, looking at a paper that, using this setup, claimed long-term memory was located in the amygdala, Lynch mocked the whole undertaking: "You would find heart cell activity increases when a rat is put back in a box where it had been shocked. Then you could write a paper called 'Aristotle Was Right: Memory Is in the Heart.'"

In the long history of the LTP debates, similar revolutionary results were found wanting for retrospectively obvious reasons. Experiments were conducted on brain slices kept at room temperature rather than body temperature; or electrical stimulations were used far beyond what was possible in actual biology. Other studies were done using immature fetal cells. These dissociated cells, grown in a dish, are far easier to manipulate than mature brain tissue. However, much of the LTP machinery is put in place as part of the cellular development and maturation process and thus by definition is absent in immature cells. "Why do people absolutely ignore the obvious fact that maturation totally rewrites the book?" asks Lynch.

> Take BDNF [a protein that helps neurons stay healthy]. Put it on dissociated neurons, and spines jump around like crazy. Put it on adult slices, and the synapses act like nothing is there. All those people using fetal cells trying to explain how BDNF affects LTP in the adult brain came up with exactly squat. Is [using immature cells] a consensus scientific judgment, or is it Jacques Derrida?

Lynch implied that social context rather than scientific merit drove much of neuroscience.

The fact is that the interesting stuff is in adults, and the cool methods are in dissociated immature neurons. And sadly, these two are far, far apart. But the hip guys have decided to ignore the distance and go where the latest, bestest techniques can be used. So most neuroscience goes nowhere. So here is the unkind remark, the traitorous comment: these agreements arise from the intense social pressures and little more. Worse still, the pertinent social structures are crude, hardly worthy of the hyperbright people they shape. Reality is a bitch, and methods—well that's just cash, modern life.

Even when mistaken ideas were disproven, their promoters skipped away unblemished. Lynch complained, often too loudly. If there had been any doubt about his relationship to those in the ruling social hierarchies, the quantal analysis debate clarified it—he didn't like them, and they didn't care much for him, either.

It wasn't solely, or even especially, the quantal analysis promoted by Tsien and Stevens that bothered Lynch. A revolution that had been building for thirty years had swept over the life sciences in the 1980s. Francis Crick and James Watson's 1953 discovery of the structure of deoxyribonucleic acid (DNA) was not merely an intellectual achievement; it had tremendous technical implications, pointing the way toward techniques by which the fundamental genetic composition of living things could be determined and rearranged.

DNA is composed of strings of nucleic acids. If unraveled, a single strand of human DNA would be about seven feet long. Each strand contains 3 billion nucleic acid pairs. Sections of these strands, varying in length from a few dozen to several thousand "base pairs," form genes. The 25,000 or so human genes make up less than a tenth of the DNA. The rest is so-called junk, perhaps a vestige of earlier evolutionary needs. The genes and junk are laid out along twenty-three pairs of long molecules called chromosomes. Every cell has copies of each chromosome and hence each gene. All genes have one function—dictating the production of proteins; this is commonly expressed by saying they encode the particular protein. Proteins, once created, carry out all the work of cells and thus the body.

Twenty years after Watson and Crick's work, scientists discovered that individual genes could be combined with one another by cutting-and-pasting techniques that use enzymes as scissors and glue. This ability to customize genes, and thus the activities they dictate, is fundamentally what is meant by genetic engineering, or recombinant genetics.

Much that was said and written about these techniques in the first few years after their discovery concentrated on their mad-scientist aspects. Would new, somehow dangerous life-forms escape from laboratory benches? Would they poison the air? Take over the earth? Within a decade these fears largely receded under an onslaught of publicity that promised miracles from the new technology. Food would be abundant. Hunger would disappear. New wonder drugs would appear. A cure for cancer was just around the corner. Most of these fears and hopes went unrealized, although portions of the predictions proved accurate.

The new techniques unquestionably had a transformative effect on scientific research itself. By the mid-1980s genetic engineering had come to dominate much of laboratory science. Molecular biologists learned to copy genes, synthesize them, multiply the world's supply in minutes or hours, and knock them in and out of laboratory animals. Manipulating genes was much simpler than figuring out what they did. The most typical way to investigate gene function was to remove an identified gene from whatever organism you were studying and see what the organism did differently.

Learning and memory research was not excluded from gene hunting. The notion that genes are deeply involved in memory long predated the discovery of LTP, and though it waxed and waned, it never disappeared. The availability of these new tools gave new prominence to the idea that memory—and LTP—depended on new proteins cranked out by the gene machine in the neuron's nucleus. What genes? What proteins? No one knew. Or rather, sometimes it seemed that everyone knew. Each neurobiologist had a favorite candidate for the memory gene.

The field became enthralled by the tools of molecular biology and their ability to manipulate genes in experimental animals. It became routine to reverse-engineer laboratory mice or rats so that they were presumed to have or lack certain qualities. The constant excitement of any one week's discovery that this gene or that was involved in memory seemed to Lynch idiotic. In his view, too many neuroscientists were swinging hammers at a problem—memory—that didn't look to him like a nail.

One of the fundamental properties of LTP, and one reason it seemed such a good candidate to be the substrate of memory, was that its effects were highly selective. One synapse could be potentiated, but another one on the same dendritic branch a mere micron away would not be affected whatsoever. "That's a pretty good trick," Lynch said. "Because they're side by side. If you measure the voltage drop that comes from this guy, you'd think you've got to be affecting that guy. But you're not."

If a memory mechanism wasn't this selective, if all the synapses on a neuron, or even on a particular spine, were potentiated at once, the brain would use up its supply of potential synapses too quickly and storage capacity would be a mere fraction of what a more selective mechanism could produce. The problem with positing that LTP was dependent on genetic activity, and the protein synthesis that resulted, was that, so far as anyone knew, protein synthesis affected a cell globally. If some sort of signal were sent from the synapse down the spine, down the dendrite, back to the cell nucleus, to start cranking out protein X, how would the new protein get back to the synapse? How would it know where to go? How could it be specific to one synapse at one spine?

Lynch had made his big bet on LTP in part because it was a mechanistic hypothesis for making memories. Encoding memory was almost certainly a process of events in the brain, he thought, not a single thing. It was a machine, a molecular machine. Each small part of the machine was important not in and of itself but because it kept the machine running. Most other memory hypotheses involved identifying one or another small part—this gene or that one. You could investigate a single small part using a single type of tool suited to the task. You couldn't investigate the process with a single tool; it was too complex.

"Synthesis is a long ways off," Lynch said.

They're nowhere near knowing what the machine is, so they can't know what the machine produces. It's like a 747 crash-landed in the jungle. The monkeys are crawling all over it, having a helluva time trying to figure out what it is. . . . I look at that entire world's literature of LTP, and some guy says protein synthesis is involved in LTP. So you ask this question: "Do you mean that in a trivial sense, whereas protein synthesis is involved in everything the brain does, so therefore it's involved in LTP? Or do you mean something more than that?" And they say, "Yeah, we mean something more than that." And then your question is, "Well, what do you mean, more than that? What?" There is no answer to what. That's the end of the story.

In a fundamental way, and without actually realizing quite what the implications would be, Lynch decided he would have none of it. He felt himself becoming more and more estranged. The field's preoccupation with technique irked him. He was bothered both by the lack of rigor and by the social pecking order that seemed to support it. Lynch had always felt he was fighting uphill, that somehow everyone else had the advantage, that he was always going to be the oddball kid from the wrong family, at the wrong universities saying the wrong things to the wrong people. He had a huge chip on his shoulder and still hadn't fully absorbed the essential lesson he learned at Princeton, which was the lesson of class. He knew intellectually what it was. He could express it vividly.

> Here's the great thing about going to Princeton. I had these kids working for me. One was getting bad grades, kid named Ballantine, Pete Ballantine. I tell him he's fucking up in a major way, he's gonna get kicked out. Pete's there, and he's like, "Well, thank you, but that's not what the counselor says. The counselor says, 'Look, you're at Princeton. You wouldn't be here if you weren't smart. You've got a psychological problem. We'll get you some counseling. You'll be fine.'"
>
> Boom, this guy walks out of there thinking he's great. Here at Irvine, a kid comes here, a little Gary Jr., gets bad grades, and they go, "You know what? You're a dumb fuck, you shouldn't be here."

As well as Lynch understood the hierarchy within which neuroscience is conducted, he couldn't reconcile himself to it in practice. He was forever incensed that he was on the outside looking in, racing to catch up if he were to have any chance at all. In many ways he was waiting for somebody to come up to him and say, *You shouldn't be here. You don't belong.* Now he didn't react by trying harder to blend in, to get along. That ceased even to be an option for him. In his mind, he had done quite enough of that already. His answer now was almost comically counterproductive. He withdrew.

"I know how he feels," said Tim Tully. ". . . He's had to hack it out on his own. It's like you're thrown off the wagon in the wilderness, and you have to survive. You tend to find your friends along the way who support you, and you make it."

At the beginning of the 1990s, for reasons that were not entirely clear even to Lynch, he retreated into his Irvine lab and seldom left. He focused on his research, continued to publish voluminously, but largely absented himself from the numerous academic conferences and symposia at which neuroscience findings are presented and debated and, not insignificantly, reputations are made and maintained. He declined to meet with visiting researchers and fought, seemingly constantly, with administrators and colleagues. He made enemies of old friends and shunned new ones. Once when the department wouldn't admit a potential grad student he liked, his response was, "What do you mean, no? You fucking pygmies."

In sum, he said, after "five years of insane arguments, trench warfare . . . it got to be very hard for me to keep playing with the boys."

Few things are more punishing to an ambitious man than to be right and unappreciated, and Lynch was baffled by the lack of affirmation. In the end, he reacted as he had before: he complained bitterly, went into a sort of self-exile, and then went back to work.

CHAPTER SIX

The History of Life on Earth

THE DINOSAUR CHAPTER (ABBREVIATED) (GREATLY), 65 MILLION B.C.

The origins of human memory, according to Lynch, lie in a jungle at the tip of Mexico's Yucatán Peninsula, where the enormous Chicxulub crater is all that remains of one of the most devastating events in the planet's history. Sixty-five million years ago, in the late Cretaceous period, a very large asteroid, perhaps nine miles across, plummeted through the atmosphere and hit the earth with such force it dug a crater one hundred miles wide, initiated tidal waves, volcanoes, and hurricane-force winds, and ignited fires that destroyed as much as a quarter of the foliage on the planet.

Beyond these immediate effects, the impact raised billions of tons of dust and debris that, combined with smoke from the fires, created a cloud so large, it darkened the earth for months, perhaps years. The Cretaceous was—or had been, until that point—the age of dinosaurs, who had had the run of the planet for at least 100 million years. The dinosaurs had evolved as mainly diurnal creatures, meaning they were active during the day and becalmed at night. Whether cause or effect it's impossible to say, but dinosaurs were extremely reliant on vision. Their sense of smell was not well developed. Said Lynch: "The big meteor comes, and guess what? It's dark and cold; they're dependent on vision, and they're diurnal. They're fucked."

The dinosaurs, along with 80 percent of the animal species on Earth, died. Among those that survived were small mammals, "nocturnal" animals with much more well-developed senses of smell. If you had a good nose, the darkness didn't matter so much.

Mammals, relative to their body size, have very large brains, much bigger than other animals. Most of the increase in size is in one portion of the brain, the cerebral cortex. Among the most elementary—that is, evolutionarily old—areas of the cortex is the olfactory area, where memories of smells are encoded. It was the presence of this relatively large olfactory cortex that allowed certain mammals to survive the asteroid extinction. Human beings, the best developed of the mammals, have extraordinarily large brains. (Brain size tends to scale to body size in all animals. Birds and mammals are the exceptions, having brains several times larger than their body sizes would predict.) Lynch thinks the olfactory cortex is the model for the development of the rest of the cortex, an area of vast undifferentiated capacity, ideal for random network storage. Ideal, in other words, for memory. Here's why.

All of the senses, except for smell, are represented in the brain by what amounts to topographical maps. When you walk down the street and look at the angle of light reflecting off a copper-domed church, that signal is sent to your brain in a one-to-one correspondence to the actual thing. The copper dome is rebuilt for a moment in your head. In a sense, this process is hard-wired. If light activates certain receptors, the brain makes a map of those receptors. The same is true of touch, taste, and hearing. Sensations received through the skin are sent to the brain and rebuilt on a virtual map of your body. An interior-brain map of your tongue corresponds to the actual location of your taste buds. Sounds you hear are represented in your brain relative to where they came from.

Smell is different. As soon as odor molecules reach the receptors in your nose, a signal is sent to a switching station in your brain called the olfactory bulb. As with the other senses, this initial signal corresponds one to one to the odor receptors that were activated. But as soon as the signal is sent on to the rest of the brain, the one-to-one correspondence is thrown away, and the information loses what we might call its shape. Why would the system throw away information? If you think about it, smells don't exist in any sort of pattern. The scent of new-mown lawn isn't related in any way to the smell of a eucalyptus tree—it is not spatially up or down or to the left or right of it; space has nothing to do with it. You might, while on a walk, experience both odors simultaneously at the corner of Valley and Eighteenth Street. There is nothing relevant about where the parts of the new combined odor came from. They are random. The brain needs a way to associate random sensory inputs, in this case odors. Throwing away a natural ordering system allows the brain to connect random inputs. "Random access networks," Lynch once wrote, "enable unified perceptions of disparate ingredients."

This process amounts to a biologically more sophisticated machine for assessing the environment. Even more, it allows disparate information to be stored, assembled, and reassembled for future use. In a random access storage system, any individual part can be associated with any other part. Lynch believes the olfactory system became the model for the evolving memory system. The topographic circuits of the other sensory systems eventually give their information to the random storage networks that characterize the olfactory system. That is, they give up their spatial orientation in exchange for the ability to associate with other perceptions. They are freed from their rigid localization of sensation. In the new system, sounds can be associated with sights or smells or touch or any combination of them all. Memory can be unified.

Lynch's consideration of these ideas was little more than a hobby for him. It hadn't much relevance to any of his research until the late 1980s, when, while fighting battles on several fronts in the LTP wars, Lynch was introduced to Rick Granger, a computer scientist recently arrived in Irvine from Yale. Granger had what he thought was a fantastic neural network model based on the work of the Swiss theorist Jean Piaget.

"Flabbergasted hardly begins to describe my reaction to this," Lynch said. "I knew from some obscure course at Princeton that Piaget was total crap, and Rick's model had no neural in it, at least as seen on this particular planet. 'Son,' I says, 'no idea what goes on back there at MIT and Yale, but you needs to get yourself into a man's world. Let's put those empirically derived learning rules into a simulation.' "

Granger went to work building a computer model of a learning system incorporating what Lynch had learned about LTP, in particular the timing rules dictated by the interactions of the AMPA and NMDA receptors and theta rhythms. The LTP requirement for the opening of the dual receptors and the fact that they opened together only if they received action potentials at a specific rate effectively meant that whatever sensory information an individual took in was thrown away if the timing rules were not met. This explains, among other things, how you can walk down the street and, if your brain isn't functioning at a specific rhythm, reach the end of the block and have no idea how you got there.

Granger ran multiple simulations, using the random access storage system of the olfactory cortex as his base model. He installed a computer terminal in Lynch's office, so that Lynch could examine the results of the simulations; he issued precise rules about which keys Lynch could touch and which he could not.

"One night," Lynch recalled, "I am sitting in my trailer across from the university credit union, punching away on the machine . . . and a network using LTP rules starts making categories—and then categories of categories. There's a moment to live for."

It was astonishing. The machine—with heavy *2001: A Space*

Odyssey implications about who was really in charge here—took over. Or, more precisely, Granger's simulated network took over and began building an utterly new system. The system, remarkably, was self-organizing. It was downright spooky.

"If you take the olfactory cortex and model it biologically and realistically, and you use LTP rules, the thing automatically makes hierarchical categories," Lynch said.

In other words, it goes, animal, bird, robin in three successive iterations, without us telling it ever to do that. It just does that. The capacity of the thing is just dumbfounding. . . . It is a magnificent machine for assembling disparate things in the environment into categories and treating them as wholes and stacking categories on top of each other. It's astounding.

Fundamentally built into the circuitry of sensory-type cortex, again with random connections—built into it is the way we feel the world. You don't walk out onto the street and look up and see a car bearing down on you and say, "Oh, a Chevrolet Impala." You say, "Car." And then if you want more information, you go down the hierarchy, you take another look and another look and another look and you just go down the hierarchy using this first observation. You go through your life in thought using broad concepts, and then you go down the hierarchy.

Lynch was fond of saying that if you weren't being surprised, if you weren't learning unanticipated things, then you weren't making worthwhile discoveries. In fact, you weren't really doing science at all. The results of the neural simulations were utterly unexpected, or even imagined. Granger and Lynch had stumbled upon what seemed to be fundamental insights into a mammalian learning process that reshaped the world even as it was taking it in. If the model was correct, categorization took place inside the brain unconsciously at the neural cellular level. LTP sculpted the world even as it was being experienced. Such a system ought to multiply the storage capacity of the cortex many times, by the mere fact of making the categories.

Here's how. Suppose a novel experience requires the brain to build a network of, say, fifteen thousand synapses. Each successive similar-but-somehow-different experience will require many fewer synapses (no one knows how many), simply because of the overlaps with the prior experience. If, over a lifetime, you constantly add to that store of experiences, by the time you are forty the number of new synapses needed to encode information about a class of familiar objects (for example, automobiles) might be quite small, perhaps hundreds compared to the original thousands of encodings.

Lynch had fled psychology after graduate school, considering as deadly accurate William James's description of it as a "sad little science." But the work he and John Larson had done on the theta rhythm and Granger's computer model forced the psychology of learning back into the discussion. Lynch couldn't avoid it. He now had two sets of rules. The first was the result of a simple timing mechanism, deriving from the interaction of theta burst stimulation and the dual AMPA/NMDA receptors: two environmental cues are automatically associated with each other if and only if they arrive within the time it takes (about one-fifth of a second) for the theta bursts to open first the AMPA channel, then the NMDA channel. That coincidence is required to initiate LTP. In other words, the whole experience of cause and effect (and indeed much of the history of philosophy) seemed to be nothing more than an artifact of molecular timing.

"So I make the modest proposition," Lynch said, "that the great philosophical question, the origin of causality, is nothing but that. Is it because the universe is filled with causal relationships within that time frame? I don't think so. It's because you inherited this olfactory system from some shit-ass primate 150 million years ago.

"This is much, much more interesting than anybody knows because of this exquisite piece, this quite elegant piece of engineering," Lynch said.

> It goes like this: If I'm right in saying that fundamental basis of causality in the emotional sense is this, then that's a profound discovery, because you've now taken down to fucking potassium channels what has been a philosophically challenging issue. Is there causality in the universe? It doesn't really make a goddamned bit of difference, because there's causality in your fucking brain. And there it is—it's a potassium channel. Now that's science to me. That's what I mean by science. But I tell you, they don't. When I say "they," I mean The They. They don't. I spin my wheels going down to this level and that's what we're doing now with LTP and with the expression mechanism. But I'm extremely dubious—I mean, *dubious* hardly captures it—that They give a shit.

In fact, no one seemed to care much about the implications of Larson's theta discovery, and, reinforcing the ho-hum reaction, funding agencies refused to grant money to study it. Lynch was never able to pursue the psychological implications. But by the time Granger appeared in Irvine, James McGaugh, a colleague of Lynch's, had a contact in, of all places, the U.S. Navy, which thought neural network simulations could have national security implications. The navy funded Granger's work.

The idea that the brain automatically shapes its response to external stimuli antedates the creation of modern psychology. Immanuel Kant, in his *Critique of Judgment*, proposed that a certain kind of aesthetic pleasure derives not from any conscious appreciation of sensory inputs but from an underlying unification of those inputs that occurs unconsciously. Take, for example, a painting that people enjoy. It isn't the painting itself that they find pleasing, but the sense of completion it induces in the viewers themselves. Linda Palmer, a philosophy professor working at Carnegie Mellon in Pittsburgh and at Lynch Lab, has been building a case that Kant's hypothesis has a neural correlate. Her hypothesis is that the brain, through LTP, generates a feeling of satisfaction when new inputs are made to align with old inputs already clustered and categorized.

There had been no known mechanism by which anything like this could occur before the Granger-Lynch model. Lynch later elaborated on the model by introducing the notion that categorization effectively sculpts information as it is received. Sculpting, by definition, means not enriching but reducing the information, and this change occurs under virtually no control of the person receiving it. The concept of *filling in* (or *closure,* as it is commonly called in the literature) is generally accepted in the broader world of psychological research. The journalist and physician Atul Gawande summarizes it succinctly: "The images in our mind are extraordinarily rich. We can tell if something is liquid or solid, heavy or light, dead or alive. But the information we work from is poor—a distorted, two-dimensional transmission with entire spots missing. So the mind fills in most of the picture."

People make errors of conflation all the time when trying to recall some event. *Yes,* a witness will say, *it was a tall black man in a green sedan,* when in fact it was a white man in a blue pickup truck. Granger's automatic hierarchical structuring would seem to account for these errors. If memories are automatically sculpted, interwoven, and made to fit into prior categories even as they are being encoded, they are likely to be intermingled—sometimes wrongly—when being recalled. It would seem to be a de facto molecular explanation for human stereotyping and an insight into the power of narrative on the human imagination. Narrative is a form of categorization, taking a nearly random set of experiences and shaping them into coherence. Such coherence may be true or false; it may also be inevitable. This notion is more postmodern than postmodernism. We automatically try to fit our experiences of the world into the shape we've already built inside our heads.

The implications of this discovery are profound. Its application to, say, the theories of learning that Granger was originally trying to simulate could be dramatic. The discovery has gone nearly unnoticed: in the twenty years since it was first published (1990), the work has been cited a mere eighty-seven times in other scientific papers, and almost all of those citations are from cell biologists, not network or brain theorists. "The rest of the world never understood the idea that LTP research threatens to reduce issues that occupied the boys from Kant to Chomsky," Lynch said.

Ironically, one reason is the often rigid categorizations of which contemporary science is so fond. The insights were important to the psychology of learning and cognition, but Lynch was writing from a physiological perspective. The very biological imperative toward categorization that the discovery described likely undermined appreciation of the description. That is, psychologists who might have welcomed the insight were probably not even aware of it.

THE BIRD-BRAIN CHAPTER

Lynch was talking one day about the implications of odd features that had been built into the brain over several hundred million years of random mutation.

If you look at the brain of a fly or the brain of Eric Kandel's animal, the *Aplysia californica*—now they don't really have brains, but if you look at their nervous systems, what really strikes you right off the top is, Eric can look at this, that nervous system, he can pick out which neuron is the one that goes and does this, which one this. In your lower brain, down here, things are much more differentiated. There the neurons controlling respiration are very different. In other words, specialized adapted neurons are archaic. The evolutionarily advanced stuff is random and generalized.

People don't really have an appreciation of what that means. What it means is, this thing [the brain] is a computer, literally a computer. It's got a good computational base element, just like any other computer; it uses it over and over again. You program this piece for this function, this piece for this function. . . . It's the key to the brain, the thing's random. The key to understanding it is, ninety percent of the human brain uses the same basic circuitry, the same basic neurons. If I took out your—if I was skilled in the art—if I took out your auditory cortex and put it under a microscope, took out a piece of visual cortex and put it under a microscope, took out a piece of motor cortex and put it under a microscope, you couldn't tell them apart. It's really freaky when you stop to think about it. Vision's doing vision, audition is doing audition. They don't seem to be very similar, and yet the circuitry's [approximately] the same.

You can't deal with the world that's out there. It generalizes away from specificity, away from hardware to programming. It's an extraordinary story that really is not appreciated, that we have gone to generalization away from specificity, towards programming away from hardware. That's really a great invention. It's a great idea. And it really is true about having LTP as an encoding machine, because LTP has all these marvelous properties. We specified LTP as synaptic learning rules, put it into computers, and it does some really, really cool things. So that's great, but there's got to be a hook in there someplace. I'm agnostic. I don't believe there's a friendly god out there. There had to be a deal. So what's the deal? And this is when I began to suspect, the day it occurred to me what the deal was going to look like was the day I was hearing this guy who studies bird brains. He's saying, "You know, the bird adds twenty thousand neurons every day to his brain."

"Well," I said, "how come that parakeet doesn't have a head the size of an elephant?"

He says, "No, they're dying. They're turning over. The bird has all kinds of nuclei in there that die from one season to the next."

You know that a fish, if you cut off the front half of the cortex, he grows it back. You cut the optic tract of a frog, he grows a new one. And if you look at the brain of a reptile, it's filled with regeneration, because it's constantly growing. And they live long lives. None of that is true with mammals. You look in the brain of a mammal, and there's no sign of growth and there's no sign of regeneration. None of those things. If you want to build the whole thing on memory as opposed to evolutionary specification, meaning I'm not going to give you a special neuron for this job, don't worry about it. Meaning I'm not going to give you a special neuron for motor, a special neuron for whatever. Instead, you can use general neurons and as you grow 'em, you can train 'em.

Why don't we, why can't we, grow new branches? Why can't we grow new cells? Your memory is buried in there. If this synapse dies, that memory is gone and it's never coming back. This cell has got no special function. . . . If you had a system with specialized function, you can kill that one and replace it with another one with the same labeling. But if all you are, if your totality, is simply in synaptic strength spread across your cortex, if anybody dies, the memory goes away and it can't be replaced, because you can't bring back

the program that was there originally, the event that pro-
grammed it.

So it dawned on me: We've made a deal with the devil
here. It isn't the secret of our existence that we have so much
plasticity. It's that we have so much stability. These dendrites
have to last a lifetime. Now, if anything happens to one of
them, there is no machinery left to repair it, or replace it. You
can't get it back. Your dendrites start to shrink. Your cells
start to atrophy. That's your tough luck. You get stupid.

"Obviously," Lynch said, "this is an evolutionary add-on. At
the Nineteenth Annual Meeting of Cells, some cell stands up
and says, 'This is nuts. We need another way to handle this
stuff.' "

THE LYNCH CHAPTER

In 1978 the DNA encoding the human insulin protein was isolated and inserted into yeast cells. Yeast cells reproduce every
few hours. If some other substance can be inserted into a yeast
cell and grown with it, you can make a lot of that substance very
quickly. Genentech, a brand-new South San Francisco company,
proved this could be done with insulin and done cheaply. Genentech had been founded with a $1,000 investment in 1976.
The company sold stock to the public in 1980, two years before it
had any products whatsoever. The stock opened at $35 a share
and went to $89 in an hour. The two men who put up the origi-
nal $1,000 suddenly had stock worth $66 million. The biotech
industry was born. And its two fundamental traits—astonishing
science and astonishing fortune—were joined.

Most university scientists devote long hours for many years
and earn not a great deal of money; for them, real wealth had
never been a reasonable prospect. Now it suddenly seemed possible. As Ronald Reagan marched triumphantly on Washington,

D.C., and similarly budget-minded politicians took control of statehouses across the country, talk of academic cost-cutting was ubiquitous. To many researchers, the newly emergent biotech industry appeared as a lifeline. "All of us were getting phone calls from potential investors," one scientist said, "young people in dark suits, mostly from Wall Street."

Another scientist said he started a company whose business plan was built on a molecule called interferon, which he wasn't entirely certain even existed. "Interferon," he said, "was something you sprinkled on stockbrokers to make them give you money."

In the go-go 1980s, getting rich was as glorious a thing as you could do, and for brain scientists the straightest path to riches was through biotech. Biotech had within its brief life span already turned some well-regarded but (their peers thought) unexceptional university scientists into fabulously wealthy men. Heated debates erupted within the academy as to whether it was somehow impure to follow them. The choice was sometimes cast as being between God or Mammon; you couldn't serve both. Even for some who saw the decision as less fraught, the whole notion of going into commerce seemed somehow unwholesome.

So, of course, Lynch plunged right in. He signed on as a cofounder of one company, Synaptics, based on a single lunchtime conversation. Its goal was to reverse-engineer neurons, a hopelessly naïve ambition that went nowhere. Nonetheless, Synaptics prospered, eventually inventing the touch-pad technology used in laptop computers. Another company, Tensor, had the goal (never quite realized) of building functioning neural circuits on computer chips. That deal had one unanticipated benefit. After a particularly irritating series of arguments with his academic department, Lynch decided he could no longer share the same office building with his colleagues. Panasonic, which was funding Tensor's brain-on-a-chip work, paid for the double-wide house trailer that Lynch had hauled onto campus and set up in a parking lot. He wired the trailer into the university systems and moved his office into it.

In 1987 Lynch and two fellow UC Irvine scientists, Carl Cotman and Ralph Bradshaw, founded another biotech company called Cortex. Their stated purpose was to study a group of molecules called growth factors that seemed to have broad, positive effects on the brain. They thought, vaguely, they might be able to make drugs that mimicked or promoted the growth factors.

In truth, they had almost no idea why they had started the company. The Genentech example was powerful. The if-he-can-do-it-I-can-too feeling was palpable. One UCI brain scientist explained the allure straightforwardly as a desire to make money: "You can wear the hair shirt when you're a functioning academic, but you retire at some point. Monks get to stay with the church; we don't."

Unfortunately for Lynch and his partners, Cortex entered the market almost exactly as the big-money moment was passing. The 1987 stock market collapse virtually shuttered the capital markets for biotech. Cortex struggled, underfunded and undirected. The founders all had different research priorities and quarreled among themselves in primate-bumping contests, as Lynch termed them. The company reflected that lack of direction. "After Cortex gets launched," Lynch said, "pretty soon they start manufacturing products, and they're the best in the world in a product called fuckup."

The company floundered with little direction to its research. The growth factors the founders had intended to pursue were much more difficult targets than they had imagined. Finally, after two years of stasis and on the heels of a highly laudatory *New York Times Magazine* story about Lynch by the well-regarded science writer George Johnson, Cortex took up Lynch's favorite enzyme, calpain, as a research target. Lynch Lab did numerous experiments illustrating calpain's destructive role (remember, calpain's chief ability is destroying internal cell structures) in several medical conditions. It was thought that a drug that would block calpain could be a bonanza. The venture capitalists promoting Cortex used Johnson's story as a virtual advertising brochure; it opened doors. That an article published in a nonscientific journal had cachet in biotech venture-capital conference rooms gives some indication of why so many start-up biotech companies failed: no one understood what they were doing, least of all the capital underwriters. The calpain story allowed Cortex to raise enough money to at least keep the doors open.

One afternoon in the lab in the autumn of 1990, Lynch was reviewing a paper by a Japanese corporate research group that discussed the varying actions of drugs that were thought to have some effects on cognition. This was a fairly disreputable field at the time, and Lynch might never have seen the paper if its main author, Isao Ito, hadn't sent him a prepublication copy. Ito reported that one of the drugs, called aniracetam, which had long been hypothesized to have some vague but positive effect on memory, increased the amount of current that passed through the AMPA receptor. The finding seemed unlikely to Lynch ("There is no scientific reason to have thought that you could modify that receptor," he said), but it was striking.

Scientists had been pursuing artificial means to improve mental performance without a shred of success for hundreds of years, probably since people became aware they had mental performance. Lynch himself had once told a BBC interviewer that it might be possible to manufacture such drugs, but immediately after raising the idea, he dismissed it as science fiction. Now, ten years later, happening upon a faint suggestion of possible promise, he immediately called over to Cortex (which had its offices across town) to see if, by chance, they had any aniracetam in the freezer. They did. Lynch hung up the phone, turned to Ursula Stäubli, one of his postdocs, and said, "You're not going home tonight."

The pair of them got in Lynch's Mustang and headed down rain-clogged roads to Cortex's offices. Lynch recalled: "Driving down the freeway in the rain, I said, 'Stäubli, we gotta get on this.' She said, 'Why do you always ask me to do this? Anytime there's a project that nobody else wants to do, you stick me with it.' "

They got the drug and sped back to the lab to see if they could replicate the experiment and the effect. "That very day, that night, she runs the experiment, and, Jesus Christ, it's true," Lynch said.

Lynch was hyped and anxious. He thought everybody who saw the paper would see what he had seen. "I thought we were in a huge race," he said.

By this point Lynch had been doing LTP experiments for seventeen years. He had described some of the specific chemical pathways by which he thought LTP occurred. The aniracetam experiment told him that the LTP effect was no all-or-nothing affair—it could be modulated. From that night on Lynch was determined to figure out how.

Recall that the basic process of LTP is initiated by the release of neurotransmitters from neurons. If a neurotransmitter attaches to the AMPA receptors on a neighboring neuron, it unlocks channels into the interior of that second neuron. Once the channel opens, sodium pours in, depolarizing the cell and eventually allowing calcium to flow in through other receptors. Lynch reasoned that if LTP is the underpinning of memory and is initiated by the opening of the AMPA receptor, which lasts just milliseconds, then perhaps some failures of memory are due to inefficient operation of the receptor. What would happen, Lynch wondered, if he could devise a way to keep the AMPA channel open slightly longer? The receptor is like a gate to the interior of the neuron. If you could somehow unlock it, you might be able to increase the effects inside the target neuron. It seemed to Lynch a perfect opportunity to create a memory drug.

"This is where being a theorist as opposed to being a researcher—well, this is where being a bullshitter has its advantages," he said.

No one else was quite so sure. Lynch proposed a discovery program to Cortex, thinking the company would be eager to find a clearly defined drug target. Cortex, to his chagrin, wasn't interested. He cast about looking for somebody else to take on the project. It became a joke in the lab—*Gary wants to do drugs, Gary needs a chemist.* About six months later Lynch heard Gary Rogers, a chemist at the University of California, Santa Barbara, speak at a seminar. He was impressed and approached Rogers afterward and told him about his idea for a memory drug based on aniracetam. Rogers thought he could build a prototype with relative ease.

Aniracetam, although it had an effect on LTP, was not itself a drug candidate, Rogers said: "Any drug you put in the blood has to go through the liver before it gets anywhere else. With aniracetam, eighty percent of it is trapped in the liver."

The idea was to build off aniracetam's structure, retaining its ability to bind to the AMPA receptor. The extent of knowledge about many pharmaceutical products does not extend much, if at all, beyond their effects. Even when a drug's effects are clear, how it produces them often is a mystery, and drug discovery has been fundamentally a haphazard endeavor. The family of drugs currently used to treat depression, for example, was developed as treatment for tuberculosis. People administering the drugs in a tuberculosis sanitarium noticed they weren't having much effect on the disease but that their patients, while still sick, were a lot happier. Thus was born the multibillion-dollar antidepressant industry.

Pharmaceutical-company discovery programs have sometimes been little more than organized scavenger hunts. Scientists round up bunches of novel compounds (often by collecting samples in exotic locations) and literally sprinkle them on human tissues to see what may happen. One great selling point of biotechnology was to replace this hit-or-miss process with "rational drug discovery." Scientists would build drugs aimed at specific targets, at specific molecules in the human body. This is seldom the way it has worked in practice. "Most pharmaceuticals have no known mechanism," Rogers said. "The FDA has never required that you prove a mechanism. They don't know how it works, and they don't care."

In this case Lynch knew precisely what he wanted: a small molecule that would bind to the AMPA receptor and in doing so enhance the effect that glutamate had when it bound to the same receptor—that is, prolong the opening of a channel into the cell. Rogers's lab boss at UCSB would not approve his participation in the Lynch project, so Rogers rented bench space in a pesticide lab down the road in Carpenteria and did the work freelance on nights and weekends.

The key challenge was to make the drug more soluble so that less of it would be trapped in the liver. The mechanics of doing so were not much different from cooking. Indeed, neuroscientists often express a low regard for chemists—*He's just a chemist*, they'll say. The implication is that chemists are the line cooks, while biologists are the executive chefs. Rogers said any good organic chemist would have approached the aniracetam imitator problem in the same way. The basic chemistry of how different elements fit together is codified in what amounts to molecular recipe books. The chemist combines different ingredients according to that knowledge (the science of it) with his or her own individual insight (the art of it).

"You reverse-engineer it," Rogers said.

Look at the structure you're working with, see how it works and how you can change it. You see what building blocks are available and know what you can buy [to alter it]. From there, it's changing out one piece at a time. It's a matter of taking them, knowing how they fit together and where there's a place to put something new. Chemists are puzzle people. There are a fixed number of elements, arranged in an infinite number of patterns. You're trying to figure it out.

Aniracetam, like many pharmaceuticals, is built around a standard molecule known as a benzene ring. Benzene is a hydrocarbon, derived from petroleum. It is used often in making drugs because it provides a sturdy structure—a good scaffold, Rogers called it.

Over several weeks Rogers synthesized more than a dozen different compounds. Then he found one he thought might work. He shipped it to Lynch in Irvine.

"The minute he sent me a compound, that soon, I realized Gary was a very serious guy," Lynch said. "We ran an LTP experiment with the compound. The wave form changed. We sat there and looked at each other. 'Wooooooooooo.' That day I wrote the grant request."

Lynch sent the request to a longtime backer of another line of his research, the U.S. Air Force (which was interested in neuroscience because its airplanes had gotten too complicated for pilots to fly competently), which agreed to pay for preliminary studies. Lynch later attempted to get a larger grant for a development program from the National Institutes of Health. He recalled the exchange this way:

LYNCH: I've got this great idea for a memory-enhancing drug.

NIH: Memory drugs? Glutamate receptors? I don't believe I've heard of that before.

LYNCH: That's kind of like the point, see.

NIH: I don't know. You really should go back to your LTP stuff. You were doing so well.

Failing to open the Washington vault, Lynch again approached Cortex, which, more than a year after he had originally spoken with its executives about developing a memory drug, still had not found a clear direction of its own. The growth factors weren't going anywhere. The calpain-inhibitor program, which had secured important early financing, had fizzled. The company decided to license the memory drugs, which Lynch by then had named ampakines. It seemed straightforward, but any deal between Lynch and Cortex had to involve the university, which co-owned the ampakine patents with Lynch and Rogers. UCI, like many universities, had not yet entered the new age of entrepreneurial university science. It took another full year for Cortex and the university just to reach a licensing agreement.

THE LOST YEARS, LATE 1990S

Drug development by its nature is a cantankerous, expensive enterprise. "There are just so many ways to fail," Rogers says. Cortex had special difficulties, many of which were rooted in its tenuous finances—it never had enough money.

But other problems were inexplicable in normal corporate terms. For example, Cortex executives once traveled to New Jersey to pitch a partnership arrangement to a major pharmaceutical company. They spent the night before the meeting in Manhattan, which was forty miles away but where one of them had a favorite hotel. The next morning they piled into a stretch limo for the ride to the Big Pharma house. The limo driver got lost and pulled into a convenience store to ask directions. The limo got high-centered in the convenience store parking lot. With a deal worth potentially hundreds of millions of dollars awaiting them, the Cortex crew were trying to push a rented limousine out of a parking lot. They showed up frazzled and an hour late. They lost the deal.

Other oddities were present in the corporate offices in Irvine, where one former CEO's wife had been hired as the interior decorator. The Cortex building is a typical low-rise suburban office-park shell that could be used for anything from dental offices to telephone call centers, which is to say that the early American furnishings with which the offices were outfitted seemed hopelessly incongruent. Among other decorating choices was a painting, hung in the boardroom, of an ocean liner leaving its home port. Not a bad image for a young start-up company, casting off into the deep blue sea, right? It depends. In this case the port was in southern England, and the ship's name? *Titanic.* Even Lynch, a connoisseur of maritime history who never saw a big ship he didn't like, found the choice odd beyond measure.

The persistent lack of money led the company to jump from one quick-hit strategy to the next and, as important, from one chief executive to another. There were seven CEOs in the first nine years. The chaos bred or was fed by (who knew which?) a collection of volatile personalities. Lynch and his cofounders disagreed on direction. (In fact, the relationship between Cotman and Lynch deteriorated so much that once, when Lynch and a few friends were eating in a restaurant and Lynch spied Cotman coming through the door, he crawled on hands and knees out of the room rather than stay and speak with him. Asked whether this was true, Lynch indicated it might have happened more than once. "Which restaurant?" he asked.) The founders and the Cortex executives also fought. The executives fought among themselves and with financiers. Cortex hired Rogers. Lynch and Rogers fought. Rogers hired Lynch's postdoc, Ursula Stäubli. Stäubli and Rogers fought.

Once Cortex took on ampakines in 1993, one of Rogers's early compounds, named CX516, became the de facto lead compound for the company. In the normal course of pharmaceutical development, a potential drug, once discovered or synthesized, is subjected to numerous rounds of tests in the laboratory. These tests, which can last years, are referred to as preclinical testing.

They involve basic lab-bench examination of the compounds and, almost always, giving the drugs in various dosages to animals. The hope is that possible toxic effects will be discovered in the animal experiments, and they often are; yet, as recent experience attests, they often are not. The overwhelming majority of drug candidates never escape the lab. They prove either too toxic or else ineffective.

If a drug does pass through the lab, it enters into a testing regimen in humans called clinical trials. Most drugs that enter clinical trials never get out of them. That is, most drugs fail in the trials, either by not having the predicted effect or by posing potential harm that for some reason was not discovered during the lab tests. Animal models are useful but nowhere near perfect for predicting either efficacy or safety in humans. It is a truism in the neurological-pharmaceutical business that lots of rats and mice have been made much smarter. Unfortunately, rats don't buy drugs. "There's a thousand things that enhance memory in rats. None of them, not one, works in humans," Lynch said.

Given the fact that ampakines were intended to affect a fundamental brain function, Cortex was especially cautious with their development. Missteps in the human brain could have tragic consequences. Ampakines were intended to have the hippocampus as a primary target, and the hippocampus, when overstimulated, is prone to seizure. "You touch it, it seizes," Lynch said. That was a bright line the drugs couldn't go near.

By the time the early ampakine candidates passed the toxicology tests, Rogers was certain he could make more potent versions that would retain the safety profiles of the weaker ones. He wanted to halt development of the early candidates and wait for the new versions to pass toxicology examination. The company executives wanted to ensure they had a drug they could safely give to humans and couldn't see a reason to wait. CX516 was taken into clinical trials for human testing.

Clinical trials are divided into three broad categories. Phase I trials are purely for safety, to determine whether use of the drug has any ill effects on potential patients. Participants in Phase I trials are generally healthy people, and the trials are small, often just a couple dozen subjects.

Phase II trials are the first genuine tests of efficacy. The drugs are given to people who are members of the group for which the drug is ultimately intended. That is, they have the condition or affliction the drug is supposed to treat. After taking the drug, the subjects are examined to determine whether the drug works. Initial Phase II trials typically use fewer than one hundred people.

Phase III trials are essentially expansions of Phase II, with many more people taking the drug for longer periods of time. Phase III also involves direct comparison of the proposed drug with already approved treatments. If the new drug offers no advantages over the old, its approval is problematic.

To conduct clinical trials, pharmaceutical companies contract with independent vendors, located all over the Western world. CX516's initial Phase I safety trial was conducted in Berlin in 1994. "We're going into the brain doing stuff nobody's ever done. There was no precedent. There was not even a hint, clue, or suggestion. An awful lot of people said this was going to just blow the brain up," Lynch said. On the night the first results were obtained, the entire lab crew huddled around a speakerphone, scribbling down data that were relayed datum by datum from Berlin. Lynch immediately plunged into an analysis of the material, emerging to declare the clinicians were right—there were no adverse effects.

The first Phase II trials followed the next year. They were conducted in Stockholm by the Karolinska Institute, the place, Lynch noted, where the Nobel Prize was awarded. Positive results were announced with considerable fanfare at a news conference at the 1996 annual meeting of the Society for Neuroscience. All the world's scientific press were there to hear Lynch proclaim the new world order rapidly approaching. The degree to which academic science regarded itself as a universe apart from commerce was illustrated by the fact that Cortex's corporate officers were barred from the room as Lynch trumpeted the announcement.

Cortex's star and stock both rose on the news. But CX516 had fundamental problems. It had a very short half-life—that is, it remained in the blood for a very short time, and thus its effects were quite limited in duration. It provided a proof of principle for ampakines but little else. In a more stable corporate environment, the strategy Cortex pursued might have succeeded. But the company, which had gone public in 1995, was punished by investors when more testing of CX516 revealed the drug's very mild potency. It worked, but just barely. Cortex stock, always flighty, gave back all its gains on the news, then kept right on falling, crashing nearly to penny-stock range. In 1998 the company was delisted from the NASDAQ exchange.

"The company made a corporate mistake. We did, I'll take responsibility," Lynch said. "In thinking about it commercially, we probably should never have done that because it [CX516] was never gonna be a drug that was gonna survive with its potency. It was intentionally very mild, with an intentionally short half-life."

Cortex bought time by licensing development rights for ampakine compounds to other companies for specific regions of the globe or specific diseases, but it was a fitful existence. Lynch meanwhile had virtually stopped communicating with the formal scientific world. He refused most invitations to speak and sent grad students and postdocs to represent the lab at neuroscience meetings. He went from being one of the most public scientists in the world to one of its most hermetic. He nursed his grudges and plotted revenge. He was certain, once the basic principles had been established, that ampakines would eventually succeed: "One good thing about having this outside world there is they're another jury. You don't want to believe LTP is memory? Fine. You stay there. I'll invent a drug that enhances LTP, I'll make millions of dollars, and fuck you."

Finally, in 2002, the company hired Roger Stoll as CEO. A big, bluff man, confident in his skills and opinions, he came to Irvine as a successful, experienced, mature medical-industry executive, a member, Lynch joked, of the Big White Man's Club. He already owned a yacht and had been headed into retirement to sail it when the Cortex board of directors, of which he was a member, pressed him to take the job.

Cortex needed him more than he needed it. He had a Ph.D. in biopharmaceutics and had spent more than thirty years in the drug and medical-device industries. The first thing Stoll did was kill the CX516 program. It came two years too late, according to one investment analyst, but Stoll nonetheless was reviled within the company for putting an end to the only remotely successful project in the company's history.

"It was never going to be a drug," he said, meaning it would never be sold commercially. Even in trials it had to be administered three times a day just to maintain an effect. Stoll shifted what development resources Cortex had left to one of Rogers's successor compounds, called CX717.

"There are two measures for a drug: potency and efficacy. First, how little do you have to give to get an effect? And how big is the effect? With 717 the answer is yes/yes," Rogers said.

"It has as close to perfect a profile as you can get," Stoll said.

Stoll put in place a plan to develop drugs for orphan indications, defined by the FDA as crippling or lethal diseases that afflict small numbers of people and for which there is no real current cure. A typical successful drug-development program might take a decade from conception to approval. The FDA cuts the time in half for orphans. The orphan strategy didn't displace ampakines; it was conceived more as a last-ditch backstop to keep the company afloat in case 717 failed. The company had still more potent compounds in its cupboard—drugs Lynch said would blow the top off your head—but 717 was an almost ideal drug candidate for a cautious company: it had a long half-life, staying in the blood long enough to produce effects, but with no apparent side effects at all. Stoll rolled the dice on the one drug.

CHAPTER SEVEN

Everything Falls Apart

LYNCH LAB, JANUARY 2005

The myth of modern science—that it proceeds carefully, scrutably, incrementally, building bit by bit from rock-solid foundations to impregnable fortresses of fact—comes unraveled in contemporary neuroscience. Fortresses, entire kingdoms, of neuroscience have been built on frail premises that were swept away entirely when the next new thing came along.

A few years ago, a huge amount of effort was spent researching the then-thought-marvelous qualities of the theretofore humble molecule nitric oxide. NO, better known in the broader world as a potentially toxic gas by-product of internal combustion engines and several industrial processes and recognized as an important signaling molecule in muscle cells, suddenly emerged as a vital actor in human memory and cognition. It was championed in the pre- or postsynaptic debates as a prime candidate to be the elusive "second messenger" sending signals back to the axon terminal. *Science* magazine, as if celebrating a rock star or president, put the thing on its cover and declared it 1998's Molecule of the Year. By the end of the next year, at least as far as memory research was concerned, nitric oxide had fallen off the edge of the earth. Little of what had been claimed on its behalf turned out to be true, and few respectable neuroscientists would go near a nitric oxide experiment.

This was but one example in a long, sad tradition of a science going off the deep end and pretending it knew how to swim. There is no guarantee, Lynch liked to say, that something is important just because you happen to study it. "There's a whole city of proven neuroscience stuff that's out there beneath the waves," Lynch said. "And guess what? Your name's on some of it. You always imagine those animals out in a herd, the wildebeests, they're running along, and a lion jumps up and takes out this guy named Clyde," he said. Then the world proceeds as if Clyde never happened. "They don't talk about Clyde anymore. It's just not good form to talk about him."

Scientists in Lynch's lab and others scattered around the globe had, over three decades, established LTP as the preeminent candidate to be the process by which the neural underpinning of memory was manufactured. They had demonstrated how LTP was initiated and revealed some of the molecular details incorporated in its process. They had arrived at a rough consensus that the defining activity of LTP occurs at the synapses where neurons meet and specifically at the neurons on the postsynaptic side of these junctions. They still did not know many or even most of the details of the chemical interactions that LTP includes. More important, they still did not know for sure what if any changes LTP induces that cause a prolonged, perhaps permanent increase in the amount of current that could pass through a neural circuit. Lynch had proposed in the 1970s that the increase in current could result only from some structural changes within the neurons themselves. He had been trying to prove this hypothesis ever since.

By January 2005, just after I arrived at the lab, Lynch thought his time was at hand. He had devised a series of experiments intended to visualize the structural change he had proposed. If successful, the experiments would visualize a trace of memory; that is, make a map of the physical changes in the brain that occurred when a memory was made. If successful, the experiments would prove once and for all that LTP was not merely hypothetical but a real, physical thing. Lynch could be wrong. It would kill him, but he could be completely, utterly wrong. It was time to quit guessing. It was time to find out if he was a candidate to stand with the Nobel greats or, in the alternative, if he was Clyde.

This iteration of Lynch Lab occupied half the second floor of the building at 101 Theory Drive. Most of the space was taken up by two parallel ranks of standard stainless-steel lab benches, complete with the usual faucets, hoses, beakers, chemical stocks, pipettes, scales, reference books, old exams, and painfully young undergraduates. Lynch and the lab's senior scientists had private offices on the perimeter, but most of the experimental work of the lab was done out on the benches.

Almost all of the journal papers that issue from the lab, no matter whose name is on them, or in what order (a never-ending source of contention), are written by Lynch. His corner office is spare and clean, a high modern glass-top, metal-frame desk, a dual-monitor Mac workstation, and a few straggling potted plants along broad undraped windows that look out over that most common of southern California territorial views: parking lots. The only decorations on the walls are a single small plaque honoring him because his papers were so often cited by other scientists and a pair of large abstract paintings of brain interiors, which are mostly purple and surprisingly pleasant to look at. Except for the collection of Starbucks takeaway cups that often accumulates next to his keyboard, he is fastidious. There is almost never more than a single pen and a pad of paper on the desktop; he keeps a spray bottle of glass cleaner handy to scrub it, which he does religiously. He usually keeps a bottle of whiskey, or two, and a brace of glasses stowed among the plants. Before serving, he scrubs the glasses with the same care he applies to the desktop.

He can almost always be found there, typing, reading, and chewing on a cigar if he has one, or on a plastic cafeteria fork if he doesn't. He has a telephone on his desk, but it is often

unplugged. When he feels the press of a grant or journal dead-
line, he can go for weeks at a time without reading, much less
answering, e-mail. He has an open, almost guileless tanned face,
so helplessly expressive your first impulse is to invite him to a
poker game. He was sixty-one when I met him, and the years
were beginning to accumulate, cutting deep lines into his face.
He is about six feet tall and rail thin but for a bit of a belly, with
tangled, graying hair that has relaxed considerably from its
Charles Manson heyday. He usually dresses in high-quality,
untucked, casual clothes that Chris Gall buys for him—Calvin
Klein and Zegna shirts, Hugo Boss jeans, and well-worn English
chukka boots, which he habitually wears until they give out, at
which point he replaces them with an identical pair.

Work in the lab is assigned largely by Lynch's judgment of
who can do what. If an undergrad is capable, he will find himself
in the middle of a crucial experiment. The lab is cruel in that
way too. If someone proves unskilled or, worse, unreliable, he is
asked to leave without ceremony. The lab has changed locations
numerous times and varied in size over time, anywhere from
three dozen people to as few as six or seven. When I was there, it
was in the lower range, around a dozen regular members with
students floating in and out. It was split into several work
groups, including scientists employed by two of Lynch's biotech
companies, but physically intermingled, sharing equipment and
space.

Lynch has always drawn an off-kilter collection of researchers. The current lab—the girl lab, as he describes it—
includes a grad student who wasn't even formally assigned there,
a postdoc who was marooned by virtue of being kicked out of her
original department, and a preternaturally talented undergrad
who is hanging out in the lab while trying to decide which med
school scholarship to accept. The senior scientists, except for
one man who seldom leaves his private office, are three women,

who occupy offices at three corners of the lab that are, coinciden-tally or not, as far from one another as they can get, and who seem to speak with one another as little as possible.

Lynch for weeks had been pestering everybody in the lab about the need to get going on the experiments. Ordinarily, he spends most of his time in his office, writing and thinking. He seldom comes out into the lab; twice in a single day would be a lot. When he does appear, the interactions are typically casual, just checking in, encouraging, harassing, consulting. When things go well on the lab benches, he can be playful.

One day Laura Colgin, a postdoc, called Lynch over to her bench as he was walking by. She reported the successful results of an experiment Ted Yanagihara, an undergrad, was running. Lynch praised Yanagihara effusively. "That's great, just wonder-ful. Excellent work," he said. This sort of praise for undergradu-ates was rare. Lynch was not a doting mentor. To the contrary, he had a fearsome reputation among the students, who whispered decades-old tales of Bad Gary behavior. Yanagihara beamed.

As Lynch turned to walk away, he said to Colgin, "See, I told you he'd get something. And you said it would never work, that it was just another one of Ted's crackpot ideas."

Colgin, as vulnerable a neuroscientist as you might ever meet, blushed and loudly objected, "I never said that."

Yanagihara looked surprised. "Laura, did you really say that?" he asked.

Lynch answered for her: "She said you'd never get a thing."

Colgin sputtered demurrals. Yanagihara looked perplexed. Lynch sauntered off, giggling.

Most days, however, he wasn't nearly so lighthearted. Having been so long a resident of it, Lynch felt a proprietary stake in the LTP field and lived in dread of being scooped on discoveries. He ran through the lab every other hour, constantly, it seemed to the other scientists, wondering what the holdup was. *What's up? What are we waiting for? When can we get going? What do you mean, we can't? Why not? Where's Rex? Where's Bin?* Curt exchanges about the cause of this or that delay became common. The residents of the lab were not gushing in praise of his patience.

Much of the work in the lab ordinarily was some variation of two basic LTP experiments. One, called patch-clamp experiments, used dissociated neurons maintained in a petri dish. The experimenter, using a high-powered microscope, first isolated a single neuron, then pressed a fluid-filled electrode onto its surface, puncturing its membrane. The membrane would seal itself around the electrode, making the fluid inside the cell and inside the electrode continuous, creating a tiny electrical circuit. The experimenter could then introduce changes to the chemical composition of the cell's interior and measure what effects the changes caused on synaptic currents. This was exceptionally tedious work. Depending on which part of the brain a patch-clamp experiment addressed, clamping a single cell could take an entire day.

The more common type of experiment was the now-classic brain-slice study. This entailed placing a thin slice of a rat's hippocampus in a nutrient bath in which it stayed alive for hours after being removed from the rat. In both types of experiment, once the brain matter was deployed, one of a variety of conditions would be imposed on the cell or the slice (usually, infusing them with chemicals known to inhibit or excite certain molecular reactions). Then the slice or cell would be stimulated with a precisely timed, placed, and quantified electric impulse. Researchers would measure what happened to that impulse as it traversed known anatomical pathways in the slice or affected the single cell.

In practice, this meant people spent extraordinary amounts of time—hours at a sitting, days or weeks in succession—staring at graphical renderings of those results on computer screens. The work was not filled with obvious drama, and I marveled at the scientists' ability to sit and stare at their screens hour after hour, unmoving except for the occasional precise note written in a lab journal. Some of them could go days without saying much more than a whispered "Wow" if something worked. The lab was thus quiet—no music; no telephones; low conversations, when there were any at all.

By blocking or inviting the action of certain molecules, the scientists were trying to find out what role if any they played in the process. Almost all discoveries in neuroscience were made by this sort of cat-and-mouse play. Scientists seldom saw the things they were looking for even after they had found them. Theoretically, they could determine all of the principal agents involved in LTP by this process of elimination. But given that any one neuron had literally tens of thousands of proteins inside it, the elimination process would outlast any single scientist's career.

Lynch talked often about hating the day-to-day process of science, the actual experiments. It was easy to see why. He was at heart a synthesizer. He could hardly bear to wait for the experiments to be finished to prove what he suspected to be true. And considering that he was still trying to work out the details of an hypothesis he had published twenty years ago, some degree of impatience seemed natural. One day, explaining his distaste for lab work, Lynch said, "There is so damned much housekeeping. The problem is biology is a very horizontal science. You have this result over here, that one over there. None of it lines up." His lack of enthusiasm for working on the bench meant that he needed others who were both capable and willing to do it. No wonder he had been unhappy about the rash of vacations people had taken between Christmas and New Year's.

The person he was most unhappy with was Eniko Kramar, a postdoc neurophysiologist who was running the crucial experiment. Kramar could hardly be regarded as a slacker. She typically worked longer and harder than anyone in the lab except

Lynch. She was used to his idiosyncrasies, but even so, his current anxiety was driving everybody crazy. Kramar wished he would go on vacation so she could work in peace.

Kramar's plight illustrated many of the contradictions inherent in postdoc life. She was exceedingly grateful to have been hired in Lynch's lab. She had gone to Washington State University, which was not well-known for much beyond its agronomy programs and not at all for neuroscience. Located in the Palouse wheat country in the far southeastern corner of her home state, Wazzou (as it was called) was a faint second even in its own system to the University of Washington in Seattle. To come to Irvine and one of the premier neuroscience labs in the world was almost an end in itself. It had paid off in terms of publications. She was lead author on the reports of several important discoveries.

But in other ways it was a miserable existence. Having come relatively late to neuroscience, she was approaching a point in her career where she needed to make significant discoveries, then move on to lead her own lab or remain locked into a career of subordinate roles. She had become, like Lynch, a virtual scientific monk, paring away the other activities in her life until all that remained was the lab. Unlike Lynch, she actually had had a wide range of outside interests—family, friendships, athletics, all of which she subordinated.

Then, too, working for Lynch was not exactly a walk in the park. He was a stingy paymaster, not just with Kramar. Over the years everybody complained about how little he paid. If someone had the temerity to ask for a raise, Lynch would sometimes not talk to him or her for weeks. Postdocs in general were virtually indentured servants. By definition they were highly educated men and women, and some research associates earned as much as $80,000 per year. But most were paid less than half that for jobs that frequently required sixty- and seventy-hour workweeks and that, again almost by definition, offered little promise for the future. In other words, they were among the brightest of their undergraduate cohorts—at least as smart as the finance and business majors who went directly from university to six-figure incomes. Yet they were slaving away for what amounted to minimum wages. They were paid by the university and formally were university employees, but their jobs were tenuous, usually dependent entirely on grants secured either by themselves or by the chiefs of the labs in which they labored.

Once they joined a lab, they had limited freedom to choose what sort of work they wanted to do and they frequently received little credit for what work they did. If all of that weren't sufficient incentive, they were often in direct competition with other postdocs in similarly benighted positions. Little wonder that American research labs were increasingly staffed by foreign students. If for some reason all Chinese nationals disappeared from American neuroscience labs tonight, there would be acres of empty bench space tomorrow morning.

Kramar's friends regarded her devotion to work as just short of self-destructive. They could barely convince her to take a night off and go out to dinner. Kramar was a senior scientist in the lab and had worked on some of its major projects since coming to Irvine five years earlier. Neuroscience has within it many distinct disciplines, or tribes, as Lynch termed them, ranging from mathematicians to evolutionary biologists. Kramar was a neurophysiologist, meaning she studied the function of brain cells. Physiologists, generally, can be likened to engineers. They're practical people, interested in how stuff works. Although it seemed to her at times that the more she did, the more Lynch demanded, they were in important respects a good team. He pointed toward the stars, while she pulled him back to the ground. He gathered scattered findings into grand schematics; she was a pointillist, a technically minded bench scientist who took care not to extrapolate beyond the results on her screen.

Even those she sometimes found suspect, wondering if some mistake hadn't buoyed her with false optimism.

When Kramar returned from her brief Christmas holiday, she plunged back into the experiment, which she had been preparing since the previous summer. An awful lot of neuroscience was aimed not at trying to determine directly what happened in a particular neural activity, but at trying to devise chemical markers that would allow a means to observe and measure the activity. This search for markers meant that a great deal of what the scientists were engaged in was the building of tools to do experiments, rather than doing the experiments themselves. In fact, the very beginning of neuroscience could be dated to Cajal's use of a silver dye to discriminate among—that is, to see—neurons. The new experiment Lynch Lab was undertaking was exactly this sort of tool-building exercise. It would provide a new way of measuring results for experiments the lab had done routinely for years. Importantly, the new measurement was visual. It involved inserting a dye that would become visible only if a particular event happened. The experiments attempted to do exactly what Cajal had done—develop a way of seeing into the new-moon darkness of the brain and, with that gift of sight, examine in detail the operations of the previously invisible, and thereby incomprehensible, thing.

The experiment would use a novel staining technique developed in the lab. Previously, the lab had been restricted to measuring the current that passed through a slice and portraying the numerical data as plots on a graph. Now the scientists hoped to take similar measurements and also photograph the physical changes within the neurons that increased that current. The larger purpose was to provide a final proof of Lynch's long-standing hypothesis that LTP was the construction of neural networks underlying memory, made possible by structural changes in the neurons within those networks.

The hypothesis in summary was this: When a neuron receives a signal from the environment, or from elsewhere in the brain, an electric spike is sent down the length of its axon to its end, called the axon terminal. About a third of the time the axon terminal will then release packets of neurotransmitters, which have been stored in little pouches in the terminal, into the extracellular space. The neurotransmitters drift across the tiny gap between the axon and a dendrite of a neighboring neuron. Some of the neurotransmitter molecules by utter chance attach to a receptor on small growths called spines on the dendrite. This process is repeated at thousands of synapses thousands of times per day. LTP is initiated when pairs of spikes arrive within a fifth of a second of each other. When this happens, and neurotransmitters released by the second spike attach to receptors, a channel opens into the cell, and calcium pours through the channel, setting off a chemical cascade inside.

A key molecule in the interior cell skeleton is called actin, a structural protein. Actin is common throughout mammalian biology. In fact, it is one of the most ubiquitous proteins; and building and rebuilding interior cell cytoskeletons is one of the most common activities cells undergo. It is, among many other things, a main method by which cells move. New cytoskeletal structures can push a cell out in a given direction. Constant repetition of the rebuilding and bulging pushes the cell to move in the direction of the bulging. It crawls.

Because it is so common, actin has been studied extensively and its characteristics are well established. Inside dendritic spines, strands of actin are linked by another molecule called spectrin to form internal cell scaffolds. Once the calcium pours into the cell, it activates calpain. Calpain slices the spectrin molecules, collapsing the internal scaffold. Other proteins come along and rebuild the actin skeleton, reconfiguring the spine. Much as the outside of a house reflects the shape of the two-by-four frame beneath it, the altered actin scaffold (referred to in this new shape as "polymerized actin") changes the exterior of its cell, making it slightly squatter with more surface area. The increased area provides space for more receptors on the cell's surface. The greater the number of receptors, the greater the chance a neurotransmitter has of finding one and making a connection between the two cells the next time the axon fires. That greater probability is what causes LTP to occur.

The new technique would employ a molecule called phalloidin, which was known to bind to polymerized actin. The phalloidin could be stained with a fluorescent dye so that anything the phalloidin bound to could be located by viewing the dye. The lab had discovered the phalloidin stain almost by accident. It had been known for years that phalloidin bound to actin, but it had been assumed that the phalloidin could not penetrate through a neuron's cell membrane. One day Bin Lin, a scientist in the lab, while preparing to inject phalloidin into a single cell, noticed that some of the toxin had dripped from his probe into the space outside the cell and, of its own accord, migrated through the membrane into the cell. Upon researching the issue, he had discovered the claim that the toxin could not penetrate the membrane originated from a single paper published several years earlier and never duplicated. At that point Lynch decided to try using the phalloidin dye in slice experiments. Initial tests were positive, and the lab spent more than a year investigating how the new tool could be used.

Lynch regards LTP as a sequential, mechanistic process. He spent his first two decades of LTP work trying and finally succeeding in working out the broad categories of that process—how and when LTP is initiated. Although this took considerable time, these were the simpler problems compared to the final stage: How does it last so long? Under most conditions, cellular processes in mammalian biology can be stopped and unwound.

Memory cannot. Once encoded, a memory can last decades. That, Lynch said, is

the deepest problem. Because maybe within three weeks you've turned over what, eighty to ninety percent of your brain, but this is still here. That's the problem, see, that's what you've got to deal with. And you have to deal with the fact that it is what we call synapse specific. You can't be changing big structures in the brain and still have memory. Memory's continuous. You walk through the day. Da duh da duh da dah. If you want to, you can stop at this moment and this day. You're leaving a trace. You can do that hundreds of thousands of times a day. So this is the big one—consolidation. We're five years now in spook land, and we're coming to the end of not knowing the answer to the big, ugly, magical question . . . What are you asking for here? You're asking for a mechanism where you put a stimulus in, the stimulus is brief, and then over a period of five to ten minutes you get a shape-change, okay? And then you convert that from being a reversible shape-change to a permanent shape-change. So let's go find somebody who does that.

Several years ago [in the early 1990s] I sent a student out and said, "Your job is to find out what the boys know about assembly." That's what grad students are for. They're the cannon fodder of science. You throw them at problems that have no chance of being solved. If you think about it, and accept that there ain't much that's new under the biological sun, you come up asking how many known biological processes could match this little multidimensional hole: rapid appearance, stabilization in minutes, affects this synapse but not one that's a micron away, and possesses extraordinary persistence. These are independent dimensions. One day, the student came back and said a new thing—integrins.

The student, Pete Vanderklish, had plowed through the cell biology literature and found a perfect candidate for Lynch's hypothesis. Integrins act crucially throughout mammalian biology to tie cells down to a particular place. They fix, for example, blood cells into place so that a cut will clot. You could think of them as a kind of cellular thread. Importantly, integrins are often prompted to action by calcium, and calcium was the initiator of Lynch's hypothesized LTP-induced internal spine change. Chris Gall urged a comprehensive study of integrin functions in the brain ever since Vanderklish identified them. Lynch finally agreed, and Eni Kramar took up the project when she arrived in the lab in 2000. She discovered that integrins indeed are called to work in the brain during the final stages of LTP. Lynch eventually made integrins a key part of his investigation, at times honoring them by referring to his overriding memory hypothesis as the adhesion hypothesis.

The idea of the current experiment was that after inducing LTP with the usual electric stimulus, the dendritic spines would run through the internal restructuring process, finally resulting in the polymerized actin. The integrins would then step up for their star turn, locking the changes into place—making the change permanent, just like a memory. The phalloidin, stained with a fluorescent dye, would be injected into the slice and bind to the actin. The dye in the actin would be illuminated under a fluorescent microscope. If the actin had in fact polymerized, the researchers ought to be able to see it, even take pictures of it, giving a visual confirmation of whether and where LTP had occurred. In the process, it would also determine whether Lynch was correct in proposing that the whole physical remodeling, the actin polymerization, was the direct result of LTP induction and part of the chain that strengthened connections between neurons, those strengthened connections constituting the underpinning of memory.

When Lynch had originally proposed this sort of rapid structural change in the 1980s, many in the field were skeptical. Eventually most researchers came around to the view that some sort of structural change was required, but it was still taken more as a matter of faith than fact. Even many who believed that structural rebuilding occurred thought it required new proteins to be sent to the synapse to do it, and they spent an awful lot of time looking for those proteins. Lynch thought it would take too long for the proteins to be manufactured in the cell nucleus; for one thing, in extreme cases the cell nucleus could be a long way from the point at which the changes were occurring. Events were already under way, and Lynch thought all the material needed to complete the job was on hand. Making new proteins would take too much time. Memory, after all, was encoded almost instantaneously in the real world.

Imagine a construction crew framing a building. If the protein-synthesis believers were right, the framers would have to put down their hammers and call their office to order a delivery every time they needed a nail. Lynch proposed the crew had the nails right there in their tool pouches. This experiment was intended to provide proof.

"If that chemistry is the same chemistry I think it is, then I can literally give you a book right now. We'll change the cover title. It won't be called blood clotting, it will be called memory, but it'll be the same chemistry. See, two blood platelets come bumping along, they go along like this." He bumped his fists together.

And they're at the site of an injury. Signals are put out, they bump into each other, then they change, each platelet changes its shape. There's a period of ten or fifteen minutes where it's reversible and they can separate and go away. But after that happens, something snaps into place, and now it's permanent, you have a clot, and it will be there as long as those platelets live. It will always be there. It's permanent.

It would have been nice if it had been something really new, mysterious: "New protein discovered at Irvine; it encodes memory." But it's not going to turn out to be. Memory proves to be stabilized by the same old crap as a wound. It's a process you know works somewhere else. Cells crawl across the skin, and they stop someplace, and they anchor, and they never move again. And they can sit there for twenty years stuck to that one place. Something did that. This is what it is. Of course, it probably won't work, but that's what we're doing right now. We're in the penumbra, the shadow land. And now comes the moment of moments.

CURSE OF THE POOLS, LATE JANUARY 2005

The experiment began with the death of a rat, which Eni Kramar accomplished quickly, using a small guillotine. Almost all neurobiological research labs use animals in their work. The most obvious reason is the lack of human subjects willing to have their brains dissected. Kevin Lee, now at the University of Virginia, said the main exceptions were times of military conflict: "You know the song, 'War, what is it good for?' Well, it turns out war is really good for neurobiology." World War I, in particular, with its onslaught of new explosive weapons technology— mines, artillery, bombs—and the resultant millions of casualties had been a boon for brain science. Dealing with the injured, medical science made huge strides in determining what brain regions govern what activities by the simple if gruesome process of matching what was missing from the brain with what was missing from behavior. Those were, in effect, the good old days of brain science.

Lacking a war, Lynch Lab used rats almost exclusively as its test organisms. Other labs used mice or even simpler creatures—fruit flies, worms, and sea slugs. Using these animal models, as they were called, was a daily expression of absolute trust in evolution as a fact of human history. Genes that performed certain known functions in fruit flies were "conserved," as the scientists termed it, and did the same or similar work in humans. This was a commonplace in science laboratories. Even as debates raged in the broader society over the idea that human beings are descended from apes, the routine use of animals to model humans in biology labs around the world was an affirmation—so widely accepted it was never even stated—that human antecedents go back way past the apes to the flies and beyond.

Working alone, it took Kramar less than five minutes to decapitate (or, as she put it, sacrifice) the animal, crack open its skull, remove the brain (like an oyster popped from its shell), and separate the hippocampus from the rest of its cortex. The hippocampus is named for its likeness to a seahorse (in Greek, *hippo* means "horse" and *kampos* means "sea monster"), although in a rat it is shaped more like a quarter moon. Using a very small saw called a microtome, a miniature version of a deli slicing machine, she then shaved the hippocampus, which is not very large to begin with (in a rat, about the size of a clipping from a thick thumbnail), into five very thin sections.

The five hippocampal slices were stashed in a cup of ice, then transferred to a small, circular Plexiglas chamber (about the circumference of an ordinary lab petri dish, but perhaps twice as tall) centered on a workbench under a microscope. The chamber was fed by separate lines carrying a nutrient-rich, warm liquid and oxygen, which together kept the brain alive and in some sense functioning despite the fact that its previous owner was twitching, headless, in a plastic trash container in the next room.

The top of the plastic chamber had cutouts that allowed two very thin glass electrodes, guided by a geared device called a micromanipulator, to be precisely implanted and held in the brain slices. One electrode was used to stimulate the tissue, and one to record current. The stimulating electrode could be set to deliver currents of precise timing and duration. The whole

microscope-micromanipulator-electrodes-dish-computer apparatus was called a rig. Kramar's primary rig was in a private
office in a corner at the very rear of the laboratory. She had
another one just outside the door and sometimes ran two experiments simultaneously. She typically closed the door when she
was doing experiments and had no distractions inside. Her rig
was situated on a bench equipped with shock absorbers to prevent the rumble of a truck or car outside in the parking lot from
disturbing the queasy equilibrium of the experiment. Because
the electrical measurements had to be precise, any equipment
that might interfere with them was grounded, and connections
were shielded with aluminum foil to prevent stray signals from
intervening. With all the foil and electrical tape and ground
wires run amok, the whole affair had a kind of jerry-built, Rube
Goldberg quality.

The next step in the experiment, after the first hippocampal
slice had been placed in the dish and the electrodes were placed
in the slice, was initiating an electrical current at the rate of the
theta rhythm. The current would pass through the slice along
previously identified pathways, setting off biochemical reactions. The recording electrode measured the current as it exited
the slice. The data were fed automatically into a computer program that translated and graphed the results nearly instantaneously.

Kramar punched a key on her computer keyboard, initiated
the electric pulse, and waited, staring at her computer screen,
where the electric current exiting the slice in the dish was measured in real time. Sometimes when doing experiments on the
rig, she read papers or made notes in her lab book, but most of
the time she sat very quietly and stared. If I asked her a question
during an experiment, she would look at me, smile thinly, answer
briefly, then return her attention to the computerized graph.
The initial readouts this time were fuzzy. The recording electrode was picking up interference from elsewhere, overwhelm-

ing the readings. Kramar tried, patiently at first, to isolate and banish the interference. She spent hours looking but never found the source. The brain tissue died in the dish.

After all the months Kramar had spent planning and designing the experiment, the day's work—the intended next step on the long march—ended before it ever really got under way. Lynch wouldn't be happy and Kramar knew it, but she was more upset she had killed a rat to no good end. The seemingly random interference was the kind of thing that drove the brain scientists crazy. It wasn't enough that the complexity of the biology opposed them, they felt, every step of the way; they had to fight even to get to the biology. Kramar had run slices in this rig day in and day out for months without anything like this ever happening.

"You do the same thing every day for a year, and then one day, for no reason at all, you can't do it," she said. "It makes no sense, but you just have to come back and do it again. Nothing's ever simple. It never is. Maybe that's why Gary always says the experiment is going to fail. At some level he knows it's impossible."

The next day the interference was gone, a ghost vanished. Kramar ran the experiment, stimulating the slices, taking her readings, then infusing the slices with the phalloidin stain. It worked perfectly. Afterward she packed the slices on ice and took them down the road to Chris Gall's lab, where a technician would prep the slices and mount them on glass slides that could be examined under a fluorescent microscope. It usually took a day or two for Kramar to get her slices back.

Waiting was a killer. Lynch, to fill the time, had asked Kramar and others in the lab to help a colleague who was trying to measure the effect of early-life stress on subsequent mental acuity. The colleague had already submitted a paper to a premier journal stating that, based on observations of rats running a maze, relatively small amounts of stress early in life showed up in middle age as cognitive deficits. The journal sent the paper back saying it would be stronger if it included corroborating evidence from physiological experiments. The colleague had no expertise in physiology and asked Lynch if he would help. The timing was terrible, coming as it did right in the middle of his own crucial experiments, but he agreed, thinking the lab could knock out the work in a couple of days.

The hypothesis was intriguing. In the experiment, rats were stressed early in life by removing their mothers' bedding, upsetting her and them. This seemingly slight change in environment had measurable effects. The young rats lost weight, and stress hormones were elevated in their blood, but there was no evident change in their behavior. As they aged, they seemed to regroup. Weight was regained; stress hormone levels dropped. Then in middle age, which for a rat was just months later, memory deficits and other cognition malfunctions appeared as if out of nowhere.

The implications of the experiment were large: Early life disturbances in rats are initially upsetting but are overcome during development. Normalcy returns. Then, not long after reaching maturity, the brain doesn't work nearly as well as it ought to. Think of the social implications if this held true for humans. As usual, doing the experiments was more complicated and time-consuming than anticipated. So in addition to the delays Kramar had faced just getting her phalloidin experiment to work, she now had to wait while the lab went full-bore on the stress tests. Everybody in the lab resented the distraction.

Several days later Kramar, with her own and Lynch's great anticipation, got her mounted phalloidin brain slices back. They were worthless. There was no sign of any polymerization whatsoever. Either the experiment had failed to produce any effect on the slices at all (unlikely), or the slices had been improperly handled. When she looked at the slices under a microscope, Kramar couldn't tell which, but whatever the case, she would have to start all over.

"It's never exactly what it's supposed to be," Lynch said the next day. "You're always surprised or horrified or pleased or something. It's not what you expected. It's always a bunch of crap."

Just then Yanagihara, the undergrad who was doing ancillary experiments for Kramar's project, poked his head inside Lynch's office. "Bad news," he said. "I have a result, and it's not a good result."

As in almost all projects in the lab, Kramar's investigation had several different lines of inquiry. The main one was the phalloidin-visualization study. Almost always, though, in order to get a paper published, evidence from other avenues of attack would be required. To that end Kramar and Yanagihara were trying to determine definitively the role of integrins by using molecules called antibodies that were known to block integrins and, they hypothesized, thus block the final stage of LTP. Kramar was doing one version of this test in her slice experiments. Yanagihara was doing another, patch-clamping single cells rather than examining slices of tissue. The two different methods were consistently yielding vague or opposing results. Everybody was on edge.

This continued for the next two weeks. They were trying to use antibodies to block integrins and thus block LTP consolidation. The antibodies were inconsistent; sometimes they blocked the action, other times not. An experiment that consistently produced inconsistent results was worse than worthless. It compromised knowledge they thought they had already established. Yet from experiment to experiment they found different results.

One morning Lynch, Kramar, and Yanagihara met to discuss what was happening. Two days before, Yanagihara had gotten absolutely perfect results. The next day, nothing. "If it had come out the way we wanted it to, we'd be done," Yanagihara said.

Lynch replied: "That's a well-known problem in science. You should quit while you're ahead."

Lynch thought perhaps the antibodies were being destroyed before they could get to the integrins. Maybe enzymes that would attack the antibodies were sequestered in pools. "Some enzymes live in the cytoplasm. They're floaters. You can't really tell if your drug has gotten where it needs to go. It's the curse of pools," he said.

That was as close as any of the three of them got to an explanation. No one really knew what was happening. They offered a variety of ways to work around the problem, but these amounted to little more than to keep trying. They resolved to use different antibodies.

"Chemistry appears [changes occur], or else I'll have to think of something else. And I haven't so far been able to come up with anything," Lynch said. "It means we've got a long, long road."

"You mean we should give up on it?" Kramar asked.

"Why the fuck would I say that?" said Lynch, clearly irked.

"So we should throw out the blot experiments?" she said.

"I'm not saying anything of the kind," he said. "What the fuck are you talking about? We don't know what the source of the problem is. That doesn't mean we shouldn't try to find out. Each of these things begins to unravel to ambiguity because the complexity of the system defeats you.

"That's the trouble with biology," he said. "There are just too damned many variables."

"It's a wonder anything ever gets done," Yanagihara said.

Lynch said, "You make progress by triangulation. It's never straightforward. If you want clean results, go be a physicist."

Later that day Lynch repeated a point he often made, that biology is literally senseless. Physicists "have their moments. We don't get that. We don't even get fucking close."

Kramar persisted with the experiment, day after day, trying it over and over again. Neurophysiologists, like other people who habitually perform routine tasks that yield wildly discrepant results—think of baseball players or gamblers—become superstitious. In an attempt to ward off inconsistencies, they insist on using the same chamber, the same rig, the same everything in their work. When something goes awry, they look around to see what's different. In this case, what the scientists saw when they looked over their shoulders was me. They joked uneasily that the run of bad results was somehow the result of a heavy cloud I had dragged to the lab.

Lynch accepted the repeated failures with surprising equanimity. He'd been through worse droughts before. The Kevin Lee micrograph siege in the early 1980s had turned an entire cohort of grad students into a legion of the damned, but the legion had kept marching, and eventually it found the first rough evidence of shape-change in neurons. Lynch knew there was nothing to do now but keep going.

He amused himself with diversions. He had been shopping for a new car; his 1987 Ford Mustang was falling apart a little bit more every day outside in the parking lot. Lynch had been a drag racer as a kid, and cars, along with good whiskey and good books, were among the few physical possessions he cared much about. He wanted to buy a brand-new Chevrolet Corvette convertible, a formidable machine, but he couldn't find the model he wanted anywhere near Irvine. While everything was failing in the lab, he found that a dealership four hundred miles north, in San Jose, had the model he wanted. He and Gall caught a flight, wrote a check, hopped into the shiny new machine, and drove south, Stones blasting away on the stereo. The car stuck to the road like paint and stormed home to faculty housing that night.

Kramar took the setbacks more personally. By the end of the month, she was exhausted and did the unthinkable—she took a weekend off.

I thought, I'm not even going to show my face. When I get like that, I have to back away from everything. I went out and bought books, then sat home and read them. The antibody thing, that's a huge problem. The antibodies are the only tool we have to show the integrins are acting. We've published that at least four times already, including two major papers not even mentioning a problem.

The central dilemma confronting them, Lynch said, was the complexity of the process they were studying. Mammalian biology is full of compensatory activity. If you stop one molecule from doing its job, another might step in and do it instead. The result is, the experimenter never knows if she has blocked the activity or not. Lynch said, "There's always a chance something else is going on that you know nothing about. We're running more and more experiments on an ever smaller point."

By March, the mood in the lab had grown very dark. One day Yanagihara said to Kramar, "This is a nervous moment."

"You're nervous?" Kramar replied. "It's my career at stake."

She laughed dryly; no one laughed with her. The integrins were a crucial part of the hypothesis, and the embarrassment of having to retract previously published conclusions would be acute; moreover, Lynch had no alternate explanation. His entire research program would be in shambles. It was remarkable that so much could go so wrong all at once. Some days the electric probes were too noisy to produce reliable results. One day a computer melted, smoke rising from its innards. Programs routinely crashed. Then a day's work would be halted when a grad student couldn't make it to the lab.

"The answer is sitting there waiting for you, and you can't do anything about it because your graduate student got his car impounded," Lynch said, then went off on a long rant about the torture of academic biology. "If I never go to another meeting, get involved in another symposium, I'll be happy. I don't care if I ever train another graduate student. Don't get me wrong. I'm pleased with the way they've turned out. Lots of them have gone on to do interesting things. But I want to be done. Done. Over."

There was the occasional ray of hope.

Finally one day Yanagihara, working with the brains of young rats, got his experiment to work right and found the result he was expecting to find. "If we get it tomorrow in middle-aged rats, it's great," he said.

"If you see a garbage can flying out of the lab onto the hedge, you'll know we didn't," Kramar said.

The next day the trash cans remained inside, but only because nobody had the energy to throw them through the window. The experiment had failed again.

CHAPTER EIGHT

A Good Rain

FORGETTING, FEBRUARY 2005

Laura Colgin was another of Lynch's rescue projects. She was a gifted mathematician who was on the verge of being thrown out of her old department when Lynch wrestled her an appointment in cognitive psychology, where she completed her Ph.D. She was in some ways a throwback to an earlier era in the lab, a kind of contemporary hippie who lived up in the Santa Ana foothills with her dog.

Colgin had become intrigued by weak electric pulses that originate in the hippocampus, apparently in the same area—the dentate gyrus—that Lynch got lost in at the beginning of the LTP era. Colgin and Lynch thought the pulses might be some sort of remnant, a degraded theta wave. Unknown to them until a journal reviewer pointed it out, other researchers had reported similar frequency waves occurring elsewhere in the brain during sleep and periods of wakeful rest. They called them sharp waves. No one knew quite what the sharp waves did.

The frequency of the sharp waves was at the low end of the ideal frequency, the theta waves, at which LTP was created. Colgin wondered what effect sharp waves would have on LTP that had already been induced. Remarkably, the sharp waves wiped out LTP completely if applied before LTP consolidated. In other words, sharp waves looked like they might play a key role in memory—an erasure mechanism for new experiences. Other research indicated that sharp waves occurred mainly when the brain wasn't engaged, when it was doing very little or nothing at all. What this seemed to indicate, in Lynch's view, was that the "default position of the brain is erasure."

As counterintuitive as it seems, the idea that there would be an active forgetting mechanism right on the cusp of the mechanism that causes memory to occur makes sense. No one remembers or would want to remember everything. Walk down the block, go to the corner store, buy a cup of coffee, and go home. What of that will you want to remember? Likely very little. There has to be a way to get rid of stuff. Sharp waves—in essence, letting the mind wander—seemed a candidate to erase current experience from memory.

Colgin's sharp wave research prompted Lynch to begin a broader investigation of ordinary, non-disease-related memory decline, which had been documented in the psychology literature for decades. The general consensus was, first of all, that memory starts to decline not long after human beings reach physical maturity. You peak somewhere around twenty years of age. After that your ability to form new memories undergoes a long, slow, but inexorable downhill slide. Several studies indicate that rate of memory decline is pretty much a straight line. You lose as much ability to remember between the ages of twenty and thirty as you do between fifty and sixty. You just don't notice it.

This decline did not show up in neurobiology laboratories. Forgetfulness was largely seen as a behavioral curiosity and was not much studied as a biological phenomenon. When it was investigated, it was generally regarded less as a process itself than as the failure of the memory, or the retrieval, process. Lynch had long understood that LTP is greatly diminished in older rats, but no experimental data supported the notion of middle-aged decline. If LTP truly were the underpinning of memory, its decline should mirror that of memory.

Lynch decided to do a more systematic search for the decline. He assigned the project to a graduate student, Chris Rex, yet another Lynch Lab oddball. He'd been an art major early in his college career at the University of California, Santa Barbara, then went to work in a virtual reality lab, where he learned computer programming and data analysis. He decided he wanted to use these new skills to study behavior, which led to switching majors. He had to go back and take two years of science classes that he'd never had, but by the time he received his undergraduate degree, he had more skills than almost any comparable recent grad. He came to Irvine as a grad student under Chris Gall. He technically didn't belong to Lynch Lab; he had come to 101 Theory as part of the regular rotation among labs that grad students do. In his case, he came to learn physiology and never left. He fell in love, he said, with the direct contact to the biology he felt doing physiology experiments. "It's more like having a conversation where the challenge is really asking the right questions," he said.

He knew of Lynch, but mainly that he was famous. He took quickly to the freedom the lab allowed. "Gary's not going to train somebody. It's sink or swim," he said. He worked with Colgin, who became his mentor. In some ways, it was the typical, and perfect, Lynch Lab setup: a mathematician taught neurophysiology to an art student who wrote computer code on the side, both of them working in a neurobiology lab run by a man who had never passed a course in biology. Every once in a while Linda Palmer, the Kant scholar from the philosophy department, dropped by to run experiments. In large part, it was this lack of disciplinary boundaries that enabled the lab to function as successfully as it did for such a long time. Nothing was out-of-bounds.

Lynch had a vague idea that one reason no one had ever found LTP decline in middle-aged animals was that no one had looked in the right places. The places where they did look were largely a matter of convenience. The great majority of dendrites of a typical triangular-shaped neuron extend from the apex of the triangle. These are called apical dendrites. A much smaller but still plentiful number, called basal dendrites, extend from the base of the neuron. Almost all LTP studies were done on apical dendrites, mainly because they are easier to identify and isolate.

But Eni Kramar had previously established that LTP in the basal dendrites, while easier to encode and larger in size, tends to be less stable than on the apical. No one knew quite what to make of it then, and the line of inquiry was dropped. Lynch sent Rex off into the basal dendrites of middle-aged rats, where—wonder of wonders—Rex found distinct failure of LTP. "We got the loss of LTP in middle-aged animals, but we don't know why," Lynch said.

This time, though, given Colgin's discovery of an active forgetting process, Lynch began formulating a broader view of the forces acting on LTP. He began to see LTP as the product of an exquisitely balanced set of inputs. Some of the inputs encourage LTP; others inhibit it. Such dual-modulated, so-called homeostatic systems are common in mammalian biology. They can fail from either direction—too little incitement or too much inhibition. The brain is a particularly complicated equilibrium machine.

Lynch had known since the early 1990s that if a neuron manufactured too much of a molecule called adenosine and released it into the extracellular space, it interfered with LTP. It was a result, he said, "I pulled out of the drawer every couple of years and looked at, then put it back, not knowing what to do with it." Now he suggested Rex administer a drug known to block adenosine's function to brain slices of the middle-aged rats where the deficit had been found. After a couple of weeks of false starts, including another computer crash and some difficulty administering the adenosine blocker, Rex decided to wait until after LTP was induced to block the adenosine. Everybody else in the lab thought it a weird idea that would never work. Lynch shook his head. "Crazy kid," he said. At one a.m. on a Saturday morning in February, Rex, by blocking adenosine, erased the LTP deficit. It was completely, utterly gone. Full LTP was restored. In brain science, even many successful experiments have vague results that can be read in various ways. Seldom was anything this clear-cut.

"It should never have worked," Lynch said.

Rex grinned and shrugged his shoulders. "Pretty lucky," he said.

What Rex seemed to have discovered was a major cause—if not *the* major cause—of one of the most persistent, widespread real-world effects of aging: increasing inability to remember. And it seemed to be caused mainly by too much of a single molecule, adenosine. The brain seemed to have two systems for erasure—excess accumulation of adenosine and sharp waves.

"What you don't erase, what's left, is memory," Lynch said. "The first thing that says of the mental world that it's not what you expected is that you're acquiring information at a prodigious rate and you're erasing it at a nearly equally prodigious rate."

After weeks of repeated failures on almost every other front, Lynch was ecstatic. "You mean this crap actually works?" he said. "Aging does not occur uniformly even across a single neuron. It's an instant default explanation for memory loss. It's getting to the point where we might have to start believing we were right."

The result seemed to have dislodged some karmic plug in the universe. Things suddenly started to work. Eni Kramar's phalloidin experiment began working precisely as planned, and her results were almost too good to be true. Typically, in experiments of this kind, getting a result once and once only is almost worse than not getting it at all. If you can't replicate the result, it's worthless. Scientists usually spend much more time replicating results than obtaining them initially. Building *n*, they call it, *n* being the common scientific abbreviation for number, or amount, of replications. (This process is noncontroversial, almost common sense, but scientists are forever being seduced by a spectacular result that can't be repeated. I once heard a scientist explain the allure this way: "I'm sitting in my lab, and a pig flies by the window. That's an *n* of 1. But by God, I'm now convinced pigs can fly.") In this case Kramar, still shaken by the last bleak months, repeated the experiment over and over. She changed manipulations, coming at the result from every direction she could think of.

"The data are perfect," Lynch said.

> I have to say I'm flabbergasted. . . . I genuinely believe that what we're staring at is the exact thing that occurs in adult mammals as they lay down memories. The exact thing. That's it. That's what I wanted. I wanted to see the thing itself. Been trying to get here since '84. I know I'm the commander of this joint and I'm going to say it's too perfect. But this is it. We've got this thing. It fits. If that result is correct, we're staring at the thing itself. It's just colossal. It's a very hard thing to believe.

Kramar was not ready to proclaim victory, but she seemed to sense it was at hand. She spent hours alone in the imaging room, studying her results, almost as if she were afraid to believe what she was seeing. She produced stunning images showing the cellular reorganization Lynch had hypothesized as the end stage of LTP. She could make it appear or disappear at will, depending on her intent.

She did a series of experiments to block LTP, and the cellular reorganization disappeared. She incorporated Rex's adenosine findings. The results were clear. Adenosine blocked the reorganization; take it away, and the process worked perfectly. She blocked the integrins; the LTP disappeared. The kindness of the science gods was cruel but welcome. Every crank of the wheel churned out another supporting result.

INSIDE LYNCH'S BRAIN, LATE FEBRUARY 2005

One morning not long afterward, Lynch woke up and could barely get out of bed. He had no balance. He could hardly walk down the hall without tipping over. This was, at first, stupidly irritating. Then it became massively worrisome. A neuroscientist who can't keep from falling over isn't much good to anyone. Within days Lynch developed an acute respiratory infection. Then, an unrelated ancient ailment involving his spine recurred, and he had an attack of gout. It was like a sick illustration of his constant complaint that you never knew what was going to go wrong next.

It got so bad, Lynch did the unthinkable—he went to see a doctor, who ordered an MRI of his brain. So Lynch, early on a sunny southern California morning, drove a few miles north to an office park in Huntington Beach and stuck his head inside a magnetic resonance imaging machine for half an hour while the machine constructed pictures of the inside of his skull. In a typical MRI each image is a very thin slice of whatever body part is in the crosshairs of the machine. A brain MRI produces in digital form what you would get if you were somehow able to take a very large kitchen mandoline and work your way down, slice by slice, from the top of a skull to the bottom. The resulting stack presents a digital photo album of the inside of the head. The idea that someone else was going to look at his head and tell him why it wasn't working offended Lynch. After the exam he asked for and received a copy of the images.

His lack of balance was thought to be the result of a viral infection of the inner ear; the MRI had been prescribed as a way to rule out other problems deeper inside. So he left the imaging clinic that day with two heads, the one with the tousled, curly gray hair, and the other bit-imaged on a CD-ROM in the pocket of his black cotton Zegna jacket. He hopped in his cobalt-blue, 400-horse Corvette convertible and headed back to the lab.

Lynch is a torque man. He drives very fast, especially in the lower gears, where the experience of speed is loud and visceral. Unless he's on the freeway, he seldom gets out of third gear. In the Corvette, third gear can mean flying blind at a hundred miles an hour down an alley. That day he was on the freeway, radio blasting, brain failing, unable to walk, head in his jacket pocket, flying south on I-5, giggling like a schoolgirl all the way.

Lynch took the CD-ROM back to his Irvine lab, where he fed the images into a computer program that allowed him to scroll from top to bottom—like riding the Magic School Bus with Ms. Frizzle—through his brain. Upon his first sight of the inside of his own head, the giggling stopped. Lynch grew uncharacteristically somber. He began to make some not altogether happy noises. There were low whistles, smacked lips, and much muttering. He shook his head a couple of times.

An MRI, as fascinating and useful as the technology can be, remains a relatively crude tool. It allows one to see larger structures inside the body. Unfortunately, the work of the brain occurs mainly at the microscale, which no imaging technology could yet efficiently resolve. The MRI would give Lynch a fly-over from 35,000 feet; what he really wanted was to blow down through the anatomical weeds, low to the ground in first gear in the 'Vette. Even at this relative remove, however, the MRI revealed cause for concern. The human brain contains in each hemisphere large cavities—literal holes in the head—called ventricles, where cerebrospinal fluid is produced. The ventricles in Lynch's brain were enlarged, which is another way of saying his brain had shrunk. This in itself came as no surprise. It's common for shrinkage to occur in aging brains. The crucial questions are how much ventricle expansion, and from what cause.

As he sat in his office, looking at his brain's emerging deficiencies blown up to quadruple scale on his giant Mac monitor, he exhaled, shook his head, pointed, and said, "Boy, Howdy. That doesn't look very good."

He slumped back in his chair. His neurologist had told him his expanded ventricles were probably "within normal range for old fucks. So," he said, "you better hope we come up with something on them ampakines. Normal or not, you don't want this shit."

He continued going to the lab every day. What else could he do? He couldn't stay away. Finally, on the last Friday in February, he realized he'd forgotten to turn in to the National Institutes of Health crucial data supporting his request for renewing one of his main grants. The grant application had been submitted months before, and the data were long past due. Lynch was stricken. Risking the loss of an existing grant through simple inattention was almost too stupid to contemplate. It just didn't happen.

That afternoon, everybody in the lab gathered in the middle of it to celebrate the incredible recent run of good fortune. Somebody dug three bottles of Sierra Nevada Pale Ale out of a lab refrigerator (right next to a reagent), and they divided it up among a dozen or so people. With no drinking glasses at hand, they poured the beer into test tubes and tiny chemical beakers. The elements of the celebration were exceedingly humble, but the scientists were almost giddy with pride and a sense of accomplishment. Lynch, standing amid the festivities, raised his beaker in a toast:

"We do adenosine, Eni's integrin experiments. We ran the table. We ran the table. Then I realize: I forgot my grant. I forgot to send the supplemental material. I promise you, I'm the only neuroscientist in history who forgot his grant. This is a fuckup of biblical proportions. Even I have to say it—that's a fuckup. This grant is cursed. It doesn't matter. I can barely walk a straight line, and I blew my grant. I'm a chronic fuckup. Who cares?" He paused, raised both hands above his head, and looked skyward. "Who cares? I have this beautiful science raining down all around me."

Lynch stood there, swaying back and forth. His face, expressive even when becalmed, now seemed about to stretch beyond the bones beneath it. His jaw worked slowly from side to side, his smile shifting with it. Spring, if it ever really leaves, comes early to southern California. That afternoon was full of its outrageous glory. The sunlight slanted in, casting a golden glow on the stainless steel and linoleum of the normally sterile lab. Lynch leaned on a lab bench for support, to keep from falling over. He stood there with his little beaker of Pale Ale and grinned his lopsided little boy's grin. He stood there like that, happy and quiet and swaying, for a long time.

CHAPTER NINE

A Magic Potion

REGROUPING, SPRING 2005

Later Lynch reflected on the run of good results:

> The experiment you're seeing in there will blow away the world. Guess what? The juggernaut is forming, and I'm part of it. I'm not having to go out there, eyes bulging, vessels popping, doing the Gary thing, saying, "What's that you just asked me? What's actin?" This time there's a whole world full of people who are now moving toward this model. And they're not moving to it because of any deep intellectual understanding. They're moving to it because of technology. The method that we've invented in there, anybody can do at home without parental supervision. It is child's play for something that previously was incredibly difficult. This time they're all going to be going the same direction. This will be a moment when all the tribes of neuroscience come to the same campfire.

He was wrong—utterly. There was no reaction. Nothing. Initially, he couldn't even get a short paper on Eniko Kramar's crucial experiment published. All the tribes were not at the same campfire. Many apparently hadn't yet learned that fire had been discovered.

When an author submits a paper to a scientific journal, the journal editors send it out for review to a panel of scientists in the relevant academic discipline. This is what is meant by peer review. It is a backbone of contemporary scientific legitimacy and is lauded by everyone involved. It is also an open opportunity for misunderstanding and mischief. The potential for problems is especially high in neuroscience, a broad field incorporating a great many distinct disciplines. Most scientists working in neuroscience aren't literally peers. If a paper is primarily based on physiological experiments and the reviewers are molecular biologists, they may not even be able to read it. If they can, they will ask why it doesn't include molecular-biological evidence.

Worse, although the paper's author doesn't know the reviewers' identities, the reviewers know the author's, and a paper can go for review to competitors who for whatever reason will not treat it fairly.

Lynch's history of antagonizing his peers sometimes made peer review of his lab's papers resemble a gauntlet more than a critique. The key to publishing (assuming the science in a paper is worthwhile) is to get a paper into the hands of the right reviewers, those both knowledgeable and objective. The reviews on Kramar's paper seemed not to even acknowledge its main point, that the lab had for the first time demonstrated, and illustrated, the physical reorganization of cells that occurs in the final stages of long-term potentiation.

One of the reviewers, in recommending against publication, complained that the scientists had looked only at a specific set of synapses, which was inexplicable as criticism. They looked there because that's where they were doing the experiment, that was where the condition they were examining existed. It would be as if a traffic engineer, having proposed adding carpool lanes to relieve congestion on the San Diego Freeway, were asked why he hadn't examined traffic patterns in Barstow.

"He might as well have said, 'Did you put up the lead shield to block the cosmic rays?' " Lynch said.

"The reviewers were obviously molecular cell biologists. They simply don't grasp what we're doing," Kramar said.

Lynch was irate, and for a couple of days after the rejection everybody avoided him. Then one morning, when I walked into his office, he was at his desk, smirking like a little boy who had emptied the cookie jar and, despite the crumbs on his cheeks, gotten away clean.

What? I asked. What happened?

"I can't tell you," he said, his grin growing.

But, of course, it was Lynch, whose capacity to conceal anything was virtually nonexistent; he had to tell. He invited me to come around behind his desk and look at his computer monitor. It displayed information on a company called Memory Pharmaceuticals, which had been founded by Eric Kandel and was a competitor of Lynch's company, Cortex.

"I'm shorting Eric's stock," Lynch cackled.

Kandel's company hadn't had much more success than Lynch's; but the same could be said of any company that had tried to manufacture drugs aimed at improving memory or any cognitive activity. As Lynch liked to say, "It's hard to fix it if you don't know how it works." Kandel put it this way: "You must realize that we're attacking the most difficult problem in all of science, the understanding of the human mind. When I entered the field, we didn't know a fucking thing about it."

They were beginning to get closer. By early 2005 Cortex's lead candidate, CX717, had sailed through Phase I initial safety trials, and the company was now applying to the FDA to conduct separate Phase II trials for its effects on sleep deprivation, Alzheimer's disease, and attention deficit hyperactivity disorder. The trials would likely be do-or-die events for Cortex, which lacked the resources to weather another series of defeats. Either the ampakine would work on one or more of the indications, in which case Lynch, Cortex, and its stock would all soar; or the company would go under. As Kandel said, "Getting drugs into trials was the easy part. Getting them out was hard."

CX717 was a more viable compound than its predecessors mainly because it had a longer half-life—that is, it stayed in the bloodstream longer and so had more opportunity to have an effect. Still other versions of the drug, developed by Gary Rogers at Cortex, were more potent simply by having a much greater effect immediately. These were referred to within the company as high-impact ampakines. Rogers struggled to develop a version that had the greater initial potency, a long half-life, and was safe to take. That problem had been an obstacle for the ampakine program almost from inception. The drugs that lacked any one of those attributes were regarded as less viable. It was, as Rogers said, a puzzle, one he had yet to solve.

Beyond paying for the FDA-mandated trials, Cortex had little control over them; they would be designed and carried out by independent clinics, which would turn over their data to Cortex. All anybody in Irvine could do was wait and try to stay sane. That CX717 was to be tested in such a variety of diseases was in part a business strategy to give Cortex as many chances of success as possible. A drug that would ameliorate any of those diseases would likely be a huge financial success.

The strategy also reflected Lynch's belief that LTP is a fundamental brain process. The ampakines' main effect is to increase signaling at synapses in the brain by prolonging the opening during LTP of the AMPA receptor channel into the neuron. The channel normally remains open for two milliseconds (two one-thousandths of a second). The drug, once it attaches to the AMPA receptor, keeps the channel open for an additional half millisecond. The theory underlying the drug was that since LTP is a probabilistic event (you can never guarantee when or at what neurons it will occur) that depends on the coincidental opening of both the AMPA and the NMDA receptors, increasing the time the AMPA receptor is open by

25 percent will increase the chance of LTP occurring by the same amount.

"Drugs that you're familiar with, psychoactive drugs, are working on systems, turning up the gain and turning down the gain, with really very broad-based effects, working on the power supplies, not inside the chips and the wiring. They don't do that. They change it globally," Lynch said.

> You take the selective serotonin reuptake inhibitor [for example, Prozac]. Great class of drugs. It's acting on one transmitter system. There's maybe a hundred thousand of these neurons in the brain. What we're talking about is all ten billion. That hasn't been on the table before . . . that's probably been lost in the shuffle. People say we've always had drugs that affect brain activity, blah, blah, blah. Yeah, we've got a drug Nembutal—it'll put you to sleep. Or speed, which will make you go faster. But they're not really reaching inside.

Whatever the cause of many neurological diseases, poor communication among neurons is almost always one of the results. Alzheimer's, for example, is thought by many researchers to be caused by the buildup of neurofibrillary tangles or amyloid plaque or both in the brain. Literally hundreds of billions of dollars have been spent to develop treatments directed at these targets, but they have been unsuccessful. Some drugs developed to stop formation of the amyloid plaques, in fact, have proven fatal. "That's a double whammy for you," Lynch said. "Your drug doesn't work, and it kills your patients."

Ampakines theoretically avoid such complications because they don't do anything the healthy brain doesn't do without them. They are intended to simply do it better. Julie Lauterborn, working in Chris Gall's lab, discovered several years earlier that some ampakine variants affected the production of compounds known as neurotrophins. These molecules, in particular brain-derived neurotrophic factor (BDNF), are essential to the maintenance of brain health and function. In fact, so many claims have been made for BDNF over the years that Lynch tended to disregard it as yet another neuroscience fad and almost certainly mistaken. He mocked the reports, often referring to the molecule as the Big Deal Growth Factor. "That's the story—everything that's wrong with the brain, BDNF will fix it," Lynch said. "To me, it was ludicrous."

Lynch's inattention to BDNF was irritating to Gall, who had established her reputation early in her career for the discovery that trophic factors are, at least in part, governed by behavior. That is, mental activity increases the production of molecules that are thought to enhance mental activity. This is the notion that underlies so many pop-psychological claims that this activity or that—listening to Mozart, playing Sudoku—will make a person smarter. Gall hadn't made any of those sorts of claims, but she had over time done extended studies of trophins. She could never get Lynch to take any of it seriously. This annoyed her more than just a little:

> It's like he's saying, "It's nice for Chris to have her own little independent thing. That way I don't have to worry about her career. She can publish on that trophic factor crap." Gary never wanted to do anything [with it]. I'm living with Mr. LTP, and he won't stimulate a goddamn rat because he doesn't care about our trophins. So everybody else in the world did that first.

That Gall could relate this story with equanimity is a testament to her personality—she has a quizzical view of the world and accepts its contradictions more as matters of curiosity than as affronts—and to the decades she and Lynch have been together. He irritates her. Of course he does—he irritates everyone. But Gall sees it as the cost of doing business with someone so brilliant. He is, after all, usually right, and their scientific collaboration has benefited both, a fact she and Lynch both make clear.

The Gall-Lynch relationship provoked surprisingly little comment in either of their labs. This was due in part to its duration, beginning when Gall was a postdoc in the 1970s, the only girl in the boy lab. She held her own by merit. She made her trophic factor discoveries while doing a postdoc in New York, then returned to Irvine as a faculty member. Although their areas of study overlapped substantially, she and Lynch were in different academic departments. She had an appointment in the medical school, and her relationship with the university was almost the opposite of his. She is a team player. The same is true in the broader scientific world: she is active in the Society for Neuroscience, which Lynch regards as a massive waste of time and does his best to disdain. Watching them work together, you could hardly tell they had any relationship at all. "If I didn't know it, I'd never guess," said Chris Rex. "You never see them give each other that look."

Lynch and Gall live in university-subsidized faculty housing on campus, about a mile up the hill from their labs. They retired the mortgage on the pleasant, 1970s-style, split-level home years before. They have no children, have generally inexpensive tastes in food and clothing, and have more money than they know what to do with. Lynch, as a result of his various forays into the business world, has become, at least by university professor standards, very rich. His founder's stock in Synaptics, the touch-pad company, would all by itself finance a comfortable retirement. Gall typically banked her entire paycheck and would sometimes go for months without looking to see how much money she had in her checking account. Whenever she did look, she often found an appallingly large amount sitting in a non-interest-bearing account. Lynch was much more engaged with his money, but his involvement was more sport than concern.

Until Lynch bought his Corvette, both drove cars that were nearly twenty years old. Lynch's car, in particular, was a mess. The first time he and I were to go to lunch together, he walked out of 101 Theory and approached the driver's side of a huge shiny black SUV in the parking lot. I was taken aback. For some reason, I hadn't envisioned him driving such a vehicle. It turned out not to be his car at all. His was the battered gray Mustang the next stall over. The driver's door on the Mustang was stuck shut, and every time Lynch got into the car, he had to enter through the passenger door and crawl across the bucket seats, somehow avoiding injury from the stick shift. The clutch was slipping on the car, too, and when Lynch put it in motion, he had to rev the engine furiously to get it to move at all. It made a hell of a racket, which he seemed not to notice.

Gall, who still drove her twenty-year-old Mustang and had been shopping for a new car almost since the day I met her, splurged instead on a personal trainer. When she and Lynch weren't working, they read or watched movies. Lynch's idea of a really good time was sitting outside somewhere in the late afternoon, preferably with the sun shining low, sipping whiskey neat. He often set his head at an angle to the sun, like a cat, luxuriating in the warmth. Without question, he had become a Californian. He had traveled to many of the world's great cities and enjoyed aspects of each, but if he had Scotch in his glass and interesting conversation, it wouldn't have made a hell of a lot of difference to him if the sun were shining on the left bank of the Seine or on "beautiful downtown Irvine."

Their vacations were usually pegged to scientific conferences or lectures they were asked to give, but Gall had developed a fondness for exploring European capitals, and the couple made at least one trip a year to the continent and another week's worth of theater in London. Lynch sometimes cut even these trips short, bailing out on engagements so he could rush back to the lab. Recently, he had spoken at a neurodegenerative disease conference in Aspen. Sparky Deadwyler, his old postdoc and barmate, also spoke there. When, after delivering their talks, they realized that bad weather was expected to move in overnight, perhaps forcing them to spend an extra day in the mountains (an opportunity others might relish), they hired a car and driver, bought a bottle of whiskey, and raced overnight through the mountains in time to catch morning flights home. More than once Lynch flew back and forth to Europe, spending less than a day on the ground in between flights.

Lynch and Gall are creatures of habit. They go to a campus Starbucks almost every morning for coffee, separate, and proceed to their respective labs. They may talk two or three times during the day and eat lunch together at a food court just off campus several times a week. At coffee and lunch they talk about work almost exclusively and often usefully. It is an opportunity to get another set of eyes on a problem, a view from another angle. Sometimes that view is literally different. Lynch's lab does mainly biochemistry and physiological experiments, measuring biochemical changes. Gall is a microscopist. Even when working on the same problem, they see things differently.

Instead of raising children, they have nurtured several generations of scientists. Really, Lynch said, look at me. Do I look like a father? "I'm too selfish. Maybe I realized that about myself at some point."

They both commonly work into the night. If they take breaks, Gall works out at her gym, Lynch at the local bar. At home Gall relaxes by watching videos or television; Lynch reads history and contemporary fiction—Pynchon, McCarthy, DeLillo—voraciously. It's difficult to name a book Lynch hasn't read and, more impressively, can't discuss at a level of detail that is frightening. He reads voluminously in history, particularly about the military, early Christianity, and the Roman Empire.

He seems not to forget any of it. In the midst of analyzing brain images, he can casually explain, for example, that the term *rostrally*, which scientists use to mean "moving forward in the brain," derives from the rostrum in the Roman Senate, a place at the front of the chamber where senators went to speak, which was itself derived from—"God, look at that," he would exclaim, interrupting himself, gesturing toward the image, then without a pause return to—the front of a ship, which might lead to a discussion of Julius Caesar crossing the Rubicon. The guy can talk.

Lynch's lack of interest in BDNF notwithstanding, Caltech and a German lab had recently reported that BDNF plays a crucial role in the LTP process. "I looked at that, and I said bullshit," Lynch said. "That's just taking one crappy body of science and joining it to another crappy body of science."

But when Eni Kramar confirmed these results to Lynch's satisfaction, the lab began to reexamine the interaction between ampakines and BDNF. What they discovered astonished Lynch. Some of the newer ampakines looked as though they could be used almost as a switch to turn on BDNF release, which then indeed boosted LTP. It would take a while to figure out how this was happening, but if the result held up, it would be like discovering a magic potion.

BDNF research and attempts to somehow get more of it delivered to the brain have had a long history. A company in San Diego went so far as to experiment with drilling holes in heads and delivering BDNF by injection. To have found a simple, apparently painless, and yet powerful means to turn on BDNF production (if that was what this turned out to be) would be a huge surprise.

Lynch was convinced that many neurological diseases—Alzheimer's, Huntington's, Parkinson's—are in part caused by the normal wear and tear that accompanies aging. Aging effects combined with specific disease malfunctions, some of them genetic in origin, lead to mental difficulties, memory loss among them, he thought. Because aging is not literally a disease but a normal fact of life, its study is not pursued with the vigor and resources devoted to diseases. Lynch thought ampakines could help ameliorate many brain diseases simply by increasing the efficiency of neuron-to-neuron signaling—in effect, compensating for aging. It wouldn't cure the diseases, but it would relieve some of the most damaging symptoms. "If we get an answer to natural brain aging, we'll get an answer to Alzheimer's," he said. "It'll fall off the table."

The first CX717 results—from a small sleep-deprivation trial conducted in England—came back in May. They were better than could have been hoped. The only drawback to the trial was its size—just sixteen men, who were deprived of a night's sleep, then given the drug and tested. Without the drug and without sleep, their test scores fell off the chart, which is a common effect of sleep deprivation: simply put, people who don't get enough sleep are cognitively handicapped. With the drug and without sleep, the subjects in the English trial tested the same as they had when well rested, and they had none of the jitteriness commonly associated with stimulants.

It was a clear win for the company. And when Cortex announced the result, its stock surged—then within weeks sank back to its previous level.

"Nobody gets this ampakine crap," Lynch said. "Drug effect one, at least as advertised on the bottle, is to increase cortical activity relative to the subcortex, and that's what they did. An awake cortex in a tired brain. More cortex, less lizard brain. Try to lift the species out of the puddle of its own crap, and what do you get?"

Lynch could joke about it, but otherwise he could do little about the lack of reaction. The other trials had yet to get under way, and too much was going on in the lab for him to brood.

The lab's run of success that had begun in February continued through the spring and summer.

TOOLS, SUMMER 2005

In science, yesterday's discoveries often become tomorrow's tools, and in mid-2005 this happened with Lynch. He thought that whatever the fate of the unpublished Kramar paper, the new method it described for visualizing the late stage of long-term potentiation was—in addition to being a valuable discovery—an important new laboratory tool. He also realized that the ampakines themselves were a tool that could be used to probe the inner workings of LTP.

Using both her visualization method and the drugs, Kramar examined the BDNF-LTP interaction, sorting out what was happening. Over the course of several months, what emerged was a picture that was at once immensely complicated and impossibly elegant.

"Endogenous BDNF does everything they said. It's all true. It's all true," Lynch said.

> But I was too lazy to read the papers carefully. Tobias Bonhoeffer [a German neuroscientist] published it. Now, Tobias has fouled off a few pitches in his time, but this time he was right. Everything is dropping into one little picture. . . . Integrin-driven actin polymerization must have positive and negative regulators. Adenosine is the negative and, that's right, fucking BDNF is its positive counterpart. *Luke, it's the good side of the Force.* It's just too cool. It needs both the integrins and the BDNF. . . . I strongly suspect that BDNF is the positive regulator of LTP consolidation, and adenosine is the negative regulator. Aging is accentuating the negative and eroding the positive. I've never seen so much stuff fall into one little box.

Through that summer and fall, almost without pause, Lynch and company steadily refined and elaborated their discoveries. Chris Rex, the grad student who had discovered LTP deficits in middle-aged rats, set up an experiment to see what would happen if he used ampakines to instigate BDNF production in those same rats. "It's a moon shot," Lynch said. "If it works, you'll never see me again."

It worked. The ampakine turned on the BDNF, and the BDNF promoted LTP. The age-related deficit disappeared. As Lynch put it later: "Middle-aged aging cured."

It was almost more than Lynch could believe. Every once in a while he would pause and shake his head. He had not gone looking for BDNF, for magic—in fact, had resisted it for years, to continue chipping away at LTP—when the magic fell out of the sky. "It's free," he'd say. "It's all free." Even Gall, the persistent BDNF advocate, was shocked.

"Now everything he does gets startlingly good results. It's amazing," she said.

I really thought that trophic factors were going to be useful and important, more for what they had conventionally been appreciated for, which is keeping tissues healthy and viable, and functioning. Actually there is a whole huge literature, which is the known literature on trophic factors, on them being protective. It isn't like diseases, degenerative diseases, happen for lack of trophic factors, but trophic factors can counteract these disease processes. So we were trying to upregulate trophic factors. Starting on the ampakines, we weren't thinking of that playing a huge role in learning or cognitive function, even though some people were saying that. I was just, "Whatever." Now, it's like really amazing, and it's almost a joke how all the different branches of what he's been doing now integrate. It's probably going to be that BDNF is tapping into the same chemistry as the integrins. It really is like a lot of things one does in a lab over time. There are some experiments, you do it and do it and do it. And you get these twenty percent effects, or "Is it statistically significant?" And you're getting results and they're interpretable. But you occasionally just nail it. You didn't know that was going to be the experiment, but you were tapping around and you hit right on the button. . . . It doesn't always work that way. People can go for years. But you do know when it hits, wow, you've nailed it, and this is a result like you've never seen a result before, and that's kind of the way results have been going.

Lynch, at Gall's persistent urging, slowly began to reintegrate himself into the wider world of science. He did a handful of press interviews. He made plans to attend a few scientific conferences. "Historically, I've blown these things off," he said, "but the new, socially integrated Lynch will be there nodding and smiling at some truly outstanding rubbish."

At the first of these meetings, in Vancouver in July, he presented the new phalloidin method and was instantly beset by offers of collaboration. "When you come back, you come back with a bang," one colleague said. The conference, and others later in 2005, had the feeling almost of a family reunion, where Lynch, the prodigal son, was welcomed back into the fold.

Many scientists profess to genuinely like going to these meetings. Younger researchers often regard attending them as a perk. It's a chance to meet people they've only read about. In the years Lynch stayed away, he sent younger members of the lab as representatives. The degree to which these largely social functions dictate one's standing in the community is evidenced by the fact that, although Lynch had continued to publish at a prodigious rate, others seemed to think he had fallen off the end of the earth. "When I first came to the lab," Chris Rex recalled, "I would go to the conferences, and people would go, 'Gary Lynch? Is he still doing science?' I got that a lot."

Unlike at, say, a convention of dentists or journalists, even the most senior scientists actually attend seminars and talks. In an unwritten protocol, they sit, often in a cluster, near the front of a room and are the most active questioners when a talk concludes. This could be exceptionally intimidating. Imagine a rising young scientist presenting his or her perhaps contrary data and looking out at a row of seats that included Tim Bliss, Graham Collingridge, Gary Lynch, and Richard Morris, all seminal figures in the field, the men who had in a large sense invented it.

Lynch was always somewhat fidgety at the meetings and amazed at what a good time other people seemed to be having. He was plotting the quickest escape back to the lab, where progress continued unabated. The progress was not without drama, however, some of it self-inflicted. Lynch continued his war with the university administration. His various fights over the years largely had been about which grad students to admit and which faculty to hire. These seemingly routine disagreements fed personality conflicts and eventually hardened into truly silly feuds. You could hardly talk to people on either side without their making juvenile comments. The catfighting had calmed somewhat when Lynch moved to 101 Theory's office park, which was physically removed from the main campus. But the move contained its own seeds of discontent. Lynch sublet a small amount of space in the lab to one of his commercial ventures. This rent was passed through directly to the university, which in the summer of 2005 decided unilaterally to increase the rent. The justification was that Lynch's companies were competing for space with the private sector, which, presumably, could afford higher rents. Except this wasn't necessarily true. The research park was almost never rented to capacity, and actual rents were much lower than what the university wanted to

charge Lynch. To add to the irony, in the fall the university honored Lynch at a black-tie dinner for his entrepreneurial successes, for translating his basic research into potential therapies.

Lynch truly hated dealing with these sorts of matters. His
typical response was passive-aggressive. He would ignore en-
treaties until it was too late, then blow up. This time the argument over money was compounded by the fact that Lynch's
ampakine patents were generating millions of dollars for the university. And they wanted still more rent money? He felt he
wasn't being treated with sufficient respect. Finally he threat-
ened to shut his lab down entirely, and to everyone's shock, this
time he followed through. He completely emptied the lab at
101 Theory. He dispersed his researchers to Gall's lab and contemplated remodeling an upstairs bedroom in his house into the
world headquarters of science. Some of his researchers were by
then—or soon would be—gone for good. Ted Yanagihara went
to med school in New York. Laura Colgin left for Europe on a
postdoc. The lab's computer expert left for private industry.
Finally Eni Kramar, whose work had launched the current run
of successes, took a job with an Irvine biotech company that had
made a lot of money with eyedrops and Botox and wanted to
establish a neuroscience program. Although she hated the timing, she worried about passing up the chance to actually make
real money for once in her life and took the job.

Lynch's health remained a problem. "Dying all the time," he
said once. "Only a matter of rate." He showed up in Vancouver
with a fever and shot full of antibiotics. He gave his lecture,
listened to others, and made small talk, all the while looking to
be on the verge of collapse. "Just to have one damned thing
that works," he said. When pressed about how he was going to
deal with his various ailments—the balance problems, the lung
problems, and whatever else happened to show up—he said:
"I put that into the Forget About It file. Don't have time to worry
about it."

Through it all he continued to write and to publish. A Lynch paper or talk is often instantly recognizable solely by its title. In a universe where papers are usually written and titled in a combination of obscure chemical symbolism and genre jargon, Lynch's papers stood out for their sometimes whimsical, often literary tone. A relatively straightforward example from the LTP literature would be: "Alterations of the GluR-B AMPA receptor subunit flip/flop expression in kainate-induced epilepsy and ischemia." Compare that to the titles of some Lynch papers: "Consolidation: A View from the Synapse," "LTP in the Eocene," "Spandrels in the Night," or "Ampakines and the Three-Fold Path to Cognitive Enhancement."

Not that this endeared Lynch to everyone in the field. In addition to the still-unpublished Kramar paper, others were rejected at a rate he had never experienced. Said Lynch: "Uneducated reviewers to the left, pygmies to right, but on came the army of science." The army's accumulating evidence was producing a rich portrait of the LTP process that seemed to have far-reaching implications. More than being a curiosity, LTP seemed to be a fundamental brain process, perhaps *the* fundamental brain process.

Lynch, almost in spite of himself, tried to fit the emerging LTP story into a bigger picture. "I need to do two things," he said.

Solidify the breakthrough, and get my arms around how big the thing is, how much of brain biology can be folded into it. We might actually be looking at—gasp—a theory of a lot. I have to meditate on it. I think when they built this thing [the human brain]—it had to be a they, it had to be a committee, cuz come on, look at it, it's a compromise, "Okay, okay, let's put EVERYTHING in" . . . I've come to suspect the change from nonmammal to mammal involved plasticity . . . dealing with a huge amount of information, self-organizing

and analyzed, all done automatically in the brain, unsupervised learning, all random. There is no reason whatsoever
Homo erectus wouldn't have gone on to rule the world just
fine. He didn't need a bigger brain. I wonder if a great deal
of what goes on with the brain is the plasticity mechanism.
And that's what you lose as you age.

Lynch began experimenting with some of the more potent,
high-impact ampakines. The effects were even more dramatic,
which was remarkable because these versions had a very short
half-life. They stayed in the blood less than an hour, but the
effect on BDNF persisted for many hours thereafter.

"You take old animals, and they're like young animals the
next day," Gall said. "The ampakine is out of their system for
like twenty hours. So it's not there anymore, and the effect
remains. So he turned an old animal into a young animal in
terms of what we think is the mechanism for learning. That is
cool. That is way cool."

CHAPTER TEN

Triumph and Disaster

THE END OF THE ARTIFACT, EARLY 2006

A disquieting aspect of LTP research was that Lynch, his colleagues, and thousands of other scientists had devoted decades to it, attempting to first understand it, then describe its details, yet all the while they had no assurance it had anything at all to do with memory. They hoped it did. Some of them believed it did. But many were unconvinced. Tim Bliss called this problem LTP's "enduring conundrum: What's it got to do with anything?"

Richard Morris, one of the leading memory researchers in England, working with Lynch in the 1980s, had executed a famous experiment in which rats were trained to find a resting platform in a pool of water, a so-called water maze of Morris's invention. When Morris used drugs to block the rats' NMDA receptors, thus preventing LTP from occurring, the rats could not remember where the platform was. That implied that NMDA receptors, a key part of the LTP mechanism, played a role in memory. Other experiments had variously implicated other parts of the LTP mechanism, so much so that Alcino Silva of UCLA thought the LTP hypothesis had been proven beyond any reasonable doubt.

"In our lab we have an objective that is at least clear," Silva said. "It may be wrong, but it's clear. We have a way of determining when we can connect two things in science. The rule we use says you can say A is connected to B when you have met four criteria." Silva's criteria were:

You have to observe B during the occurrence of A.

If you delete A, you should see B affected.

If you decrease the probability of A, you should see a decrease in the probability of B; if you increase A, you should see an increase in B.

Whatever you know about A has to be integrated with what you know about B.

"All four criteria have been met for LTP," Silva said.

This has been done. This is something that goes majorly unrecognized. If you asked me what is one of the greatest discoveries of the 1990s in neuroscience, what I would say, and although this was a gradual thing, the criteria were met slowly—what is it we know that we didn't know before—and I would say without hesitation that it is this: LTP is memory. No one believes it? It's not because of the science, it's because of the philosophy. If you cannot agree on a set of criteria that you need to demonstrate something, how can you ever agree when you get it? Because you don't recognize it. This is hampering us. If we don't know that we got to step one, how can we go to step two? We have this amazing prize, and we don't recognize it. We are in this Neverland of not having the result to go forward because we keep going back to that. I think we have this unequivocally. Think of the enormous impact of there being discovered the foundation stone of memory. This is as big as it ever gets in science. This is Einstein big. This is Newton big. The best time in science is when you have the backbone of something. Finally now we have a backbone to memory. The real fast growth, the explosion of information is coming.

The degree to which Silva was right about the lack of recognition was illustrated by the godfather himself, Eric Kandel, who in a 2006 interview said he was far from convinced LTP had any real-world significance whatsoever. "You know what LTP is? It's an artificial way of stimulating your brain in a dish," he said. "Who the fuck knows if this is what happens in learning and memory?"

That sort of pronouncement has cowed other scientists from making claims about memory and LTP. In 1984 Lynch published his landmark paper proclaiming outright a new hypothesis for "The Biochemistry of Memory," but for long stretches of his LTP research, he seldom used the word *memory* to describe its relevance. He once gave a talk to a UCLA symposium in which he repeatedly referred to LTP as a presumed "substrate of behavioral plasticity," a phrase nearly perfect in its obfuscation. Behavioral plasticity? Not even Lynch knew what that meant.

For Lynch, now that his lab had built a solid description of the LTP mechanism, the great final task would be to link LTP, the whole process, unequivocally to learning and memory. There was a chance (he thought it slim) that he had spent thirty years chasing a mere curiosity, "an interesting little piece of biology," as he put it, with no relevance beyond the lab bench. "It's no good getting there if it's not knitted into the web of science."

This worried Lynch. Well, that's a considerable understatement: it scared the hell out of him. He determined to use the new visualization method to try to show without question that LTP was memory.

The outline of Lynch's LTP hypothesis was this. When you experience a sensation in the outside world, perhaps seeing, smelling, or touching something, the sensory organs translate the sensation into an electrical signal that is routed to the brain. There it causes the neurons that receive the electrical stimulus to release chemicals to neighboring neurons. A cascade of chemical events inside those neighboring neurons results in the interior reorganization of spines on the neurons' dendrites. That reorganization, in turn, strengthens the connection between cells at the synapses. The broader hypothesis is that networks of neurons with strengthened connections constitute the biochemical underpinning of memory.

The visualization technique the lab had developed involved staining molecules inside neurons to mark the fundamental reorganization of dendritic spines. So far Lynch Lab had introduced and used the technique in normal LTP bench experiments; that is to say, they had artificially induced LTP. Lynch wanted to carry the method from the lab bench to the learning behavior of actual animals. They would train rats in a new task, something that would necessarily be encoded into memory. Then the phalloidin stain would be injected into the rats' brains, where it would (as in brain slices) attach to newly formed and polymerized strings of actin. The hypothesis was that when you later examined the rat's brain, the areas that had been stained with new actin would be the neural traces of the memory.

Scientists for more than a century had been trying to find such traces, often referred to as engrams. For a time in the mid-twentieth century, as we have seen, the search for engrams had been furious, an all-consuming but futile chase. Scientists had since all but abandoned it as a sort of pipe dream. They simply had no way to look for it. When LTP was discovered, everybody gladly put the engram search back on the shelf. When you mention engrams to contemporary neuroscientists, they often give a bemused laugh.

His goal, Lynch wrote in an e-mail, was to "use the phalloidin method to see spines encode memory in real rats after real learning. LTP meets memory, integrins/actin meet the real world. . . . Maps of memory encoding sites in the brain. The crowd goes wild!!!"

The crowd, such as it was, would need some patience. It took nearly half a year to get the experiment up and running. Part of the problem was that Lynch didn't even have a lab. He had shut down 101 Theory. Some of the scientists had left the university.

Others had moved to Chris Gall's lab, where Lynch too had moved into a spare office and where the work was to be resumed. Remarkably, Gall didn't complain about or resist the invasion. She saw it as a logical extension of the close collaboration the two labs had maintained for years. The fact that the two labs were now integrated was a matter of convenience and geography more than scientific import.

The first task of the combined labs was to demonstrate that the visualization method would work in vivo—that is, in live animals. Just finding the best way to inject the phalloidin stain took a month. Working out the rest of the protocols was equally fitful. The mood swings en route to perfecting a method are suggested in this log of Lynch e-mails:

Sept. 10: "Step one of the big method seems to have worked as of 10 minutes ago. The Götterdämmerung of LTP/memory approaches."

Sept. 22: "In vivo struggles on and I suspect will require divine intervention."

Oct. 6: "Close very close . . . all set up for the killer result."

Oct. 10: "Won't get my hoped-for grand finale on Thursday." Later that same day, when it didn't work, Lynch reported his own imminent suicide: "Blam, right through the brain stem."

Oct. 19: "Okay, so this is it . . . the exact instant. Probably wrong, certainly too early, but . . ." Later that night: "So in all its ambiguity and certain to be wrong, here it is, one rat, one control. The little bright thingies [on a photograph] are spines in a rat learning a complex new world. I don't believe any of this . . . but this is indeed what it would look like."

Oct. 26: "Of course this is about 2 rats . . . probably will never see this again. The malevolent deity law."

Nov. 3: "Theoretically, that is an image of what the animal learned. It's an engram. Now you sit here wondering, Have we actually done this thing? To think that we have is too much, but, yup, ladies and gentlemen, that's memory. . . . That actin may be a picture of a memory. It's a big one."

Dec. 7: "Actin project now has full-time graduate student driving it (like Laura Lee Colgin—been an outlaw all his life, and so winds up in the legion of the damned). Getting really good stuff and ready to move on to learning."

Dec. 11, when they finally got the protocols worked out: "There is now peace in the valley."

The next test would be to run a proper experiment, injecting rats with the phalloidin and allowing some to roam free in the T-maze and keeping others in their cages. Presumably the roaming rats would learn and remember something of their environment, then convert this learning into memories that caused more actin to polymerize. After the roaming period, the rats would be sacrificed and the brains of both the roaming rats and the caged rats would be examined for polymerized actin. This was another intermediate step. If successful, it would confirm that the method worked in living animals. Lynch's account:

Jan. 10: "Something amazing actually. We have modified the actin labeling method for in vivo use. Now have live real-time pictures of cytoskeleton assembling and disassembling at single synapses, all within 5–10 minutes. Direct visualization of the dynamic spine in the adult brain . . . Totally not what I ever expected. A constant dynamic process. It could mean nothing. Just idiotic biology with no meaning at all. This now takes me down to a level where I always wanted to get to. It's the computer itself."

Jan. 17: "The experiment will not work—and we have the first crude version—initially."

Jan. 31: "So at this instant they tell me that it's really true: exploration causes a massive increase in the number of spines with actin polymerization in exactly that place related to spatial memory. Have to wait for all the re-working, re-analysis, but this is probably it. Friday we do formal learning, or another graduate student is cast into the outer darkness." Later that day: "It's all true . . . 27 years could have ended in a highly specific bit of biology . . . and a bullet. But it didn't. Praise the Lord."

Feb. 22: "We will do the experiment tomorrow and get the results the next day. Things are closing in."

It took an extra day, but that Saturday evening, February 25, at about eight p.m., Eni Kramar, who hadn't yet left for her new job, was at the microscope comparing slides from the control animals with animals that had been trained. The difference was startling. She started screaming.

Lynch was in the bathroom at the time. Kramar entertained the idea of busting in on him but regained sanity quickly enough to wait for his return. When he did he was greeted with a roomful of researchers "yipping and yelping" and jumping around.

The next Monday Lynch gathered the group in the Gall Lab conference room to make preparations for the final push. "Now," he said, "as we come to the end of the LTP saga, the question arises again: Where are the synapses? Where do you look? Even in a rat there are a trillion or so synapses. Where are you going to look?"

He had decided that the rats would learn pairs of odors: lemon-orange, almond-anise, strawberry-chocolate, and mint-peppermint. He had over the years used odor-learning tasks several times, so he knew the olfactory anatomy of rats well. It was, he believed, evolutionarily the oldest memory system and was simpler to navigate than other sensory systems.

"The olfactory advantage is that we understand where odor

memory is encoded. We know a priori that if the animal learns, it has to be here. In the visual cortex, you don't know where to start. This is the only place in the body where dendrites encounter the world," he said, explaining that olfactory dendrites extend all the way to the interior surfaces of the nose. "There's no blood-brain barrier. That's why it works. The receptors are on the dendrites, and it's just two synapses to the cortex. . . . If there's any place where you have a realistic chance of succeeding, it's here."

Vadim Fedulov, a graduate student, was assigned to run the rats in a maze in the odor-learning experiment. He had been in the lab for just a couple of months. Lynch had agreed to take him on when it looked as if he might be tossed out of grad school altogether. He was young, very bright, somewhat unpredictable, and not punctual at all.

ADHD, SPRING 2006

On the morning of March 6, 2006, before the markets opened, Cortex announced the results of a clinical trial in which the ampakine CX717 had been given to adults diagnosed with attention deficit hyperactivity disorder (ADHD). The results were an unqualified success. The drug reduced ADHD symptoms across the board, at least equal to existing medications—mainly stimulants—without any of the stimulants' deleterious side effects.

ADHD is thought to be caused by too much or too little production of neurotransmitters. The main treatment to date has been the prescription of a stimulant such as Ritalin or Adderall, which increase or inhibit production of one or more of the neurotransmitters. The previous month an expert FDA panel had warned that these stimulants pose a risk for strokes and heart attacks and recommended a strong warning accompany sale of the drugs. The ampakine theoretically would have no such risk.

In fact, no significant side effects were uncovered in the trial at all.

Cortex stock doubled in value over the next week. CEO Roger Stoll announced the company was in negotiations with at least eight big pharmaceutical companies that wanted to license CX717. Such a deal, Stoll said, would immediately be worth as much as $30 million to the company and eventually several hundred million dollars. Stoll's earlier decision to halt Cortex's other ampakine programs and focus all the company's resources on 717 looked in retrospect as if it had saved the company.

"That's what I came here to do," he said.

Lynch was ecstatic as well. It was the first really big public demonstration of the power of the ampakines. He expected more to follow, but this was a day he had waited for for fifteen years.

"It's immensely gratifying. It really is,"he said. "It validates the principle that you can treat neurological diseases by increasing cortical communication."

Lynch, feeling magnanimous, in the next couple of weeks called a truce in his war with the university administration and moved back to the lab at 101 Theory. The crew was notably reduced. Danielle Simmons took over Eni Kramar's role directing the engram search. Fedulov built the T-maze, which was outfitted with sliding doors and flashing lights and apertures through which he inserted cotton swabs soaked in various scents and began training the rats. The engram approached.

Lynch was scheduled to speak at a pharmaceutical conference in San Francisco. He prepared his talk and also, at some level, prepared to be welcomed as a conquering hero. In early April, two days before he left for the conference, the FDA called Cortex and told the company it had found unspecified problems in preclinical results (that is, lab work) with CX717. It ordered an immediate halt to all clinical trials.

On Monday morning, when Lynch was scheduled to speak at

the conference, the clinical hold was announced to the general public. Lynch had a bronchial infection and was loaded with antibiotics and steroids; his plane was two hours late because of bad weather at SFO. Cortex stock fell 60 percent on the FDA announcement. The subject of Lynch's talk was the failure of translation from preclinical lab work to clinical trials in memory drugs. *Irony* isn't quite strong enough a word to describe the circumstance. Lynch had no objection to the FDA's action, even though he thought the hold would be resolved relatively painlessly. "They're doing what they have to do," he said. "We're putting stuff in people's brains, and they should be careful."

Lynch returned to Irvine, the lab, and the odor-learning experiment. "Could be a thrill-of-victory-agony-of-defeat day here at the wide world of science," he said in mid-April.

Fedulov had trained three rats in the odor test and was ready to inject the dye and have the brains prepared for examination. Two of the three rats, for reasons unknown, died after the injections. The sole remaining rat was sacrificed, its hippocampus sliced and set on slides. Fedulov had the slides at 101 Theory. Lynch wanted to look at them at Gall Lab, where Julie Lauterborn, an expert microscopist, could read and photograph the images. He called Fedulov and asked that he bring the slides to Gall Lab.

Tracy Shors, a neuropsychologist from Rutgers who earlier in her career had written a much-discussed paper casting a skeptical eye on the role of LTP in memory, happened to be on the UCI campus that day. She and Lynch were old friends, and they had met that morning to discuss the various researches they had been pursuing. When Lynch told her about the afternoon's prospects, she was interested but remained skeptical that LTP was anything more than a laboratory artifact. Bring me an engram, she said. Bring me an engram.

Rather than sit around waiting for Fedulov, Lynch, just about dying from anxiety, went to lunch. When he returned, Fedulov was still nowhere to be found. Neither was Chris Rex, who had proven an able interpreter between Lynch and the alien world of grad students. Rex was in class. And there was Lynch, the big experimental result waiting—no brains, no scientists. It shouldn't be this hard, he said. "You'd think I was trying to launch the space shuttle."

Lynch called Fedulov on his cell again. He'd come and gone and left the slides in a refrigerator, neglecting to tell anyone where they were. To further darken the atmosphere, a short paper Lynch had written describing the preliminary results of this work had come back from the journal editor. It had been declined with scathing reviews, reviews a first-year grad student would have been ashamed to receive.

One reviewer wrote:

It is simply not credible, as these authors claim, that the low frequency of rhodamine-phalloidin stained cells they observe reflects differences in the assembly state of the actin cytoskeleton between different neurons. Such a conclusion contradicts all the assembled cell biological knowledge of cytoskeletal function and cellular actin dynamics in particular. . . . It would be extremely misleading to the Neuroscience community to communicate the authors' claims for a relationship of their staining patterns to learning and memory. I strongly recommend against publication of this flawed work.

"All the cell biological knowledge of cytoskeletal function?" Whew! This was, in review-speak, akin to calling Lynch a third grader. Or a fake. Lynch kept reading parts of the review aloud, smacking his forehead and shouting. Further on, the reviewer wondered why Lynch had not cited a particular paper. Lynch had been unaware of the paper, but when he looked it up, it seemed nearly worthless to him. He also checked to see who else had cited the paper. It had been previously cited only once—by one of its authors, who seemed very likely to be the reviewer, and an angry one at that. Lynch was convinced that one of the other reviews, also negative, was written by a scientist with whom he had once been friendly. The friendship had ended when a graduate student of Lynch's was hired as a postdoc in the reviewer's lab and within a few months stole the reviewer's girlfriend. It was quite hard enough just doing the experiments, Lynch thought, without having to worry about whom your postdocs were bedding.

Fedulov finally showed up, retrieved the slides, and mounted the first of them in the microscope. Anticipation mounted as well. Heightening the drama, the room was darkened so that the small crowd that had gathered could view the images on the screen. One of the great difficulties in finding the markings of memory, assuming you even know what they look like, is knowing where to search. The brain, at the nanoscale, is a very big place. Even a rat has a trillion synapses. Lauterborn searched through the slides, found the olfactory cortex, and moved aside to let Lynch take a look. He immediately began oohing and ahhing. "Oh, Julie, those are going to be spines. Oh. Oh. Yes, yes, they could." He continued to scan across the slides. "Yes, yes, yes, YES. I'm almost convinced. Almost."

Lauterborn took digital photographs of the slides through the microscope and immediately brought up the images for more detailed examination. The images were practically identical to those Kramar had produced in her bench experiments—interminable fields of dull gray tissue lit up here and there, sparsely, but spectacularly, by brightly stained dendritic branches and spines. The difference now was that the images were produced in a rat's brain by the rat's interaction with the environment, by learning, not by artificial simulation.

Lynch scanned across the olfactory cortex to the hippocampus: "That's gorgeous. . . . That's the way the world's supposed to be. Look at that. Look at those spines. That's what I expected. . . . Look at that picture there. That's what it looks like after LTP. All this time, that is the picture I wanted to see. Right there."

The following week the scientists replicated the experiment with four more rats.

Lynch was back at the microscope.

"You see 'em? You see 'em? Look at them." He traced on a piece of paper the path from the nose to the point on the image we were viewing. "It's a direct connection between the olfactory cortex and the hippocampus. Four synapses from the nose to the hippocampus."

Exultant, he began ad-libbing a song to the tune of the Beatles' "Paperback Writer." "Once I was an anatomist and I looked through scopes. Now I'm just a paper writer. Paper writer." He stopped the song midstanza. "THAT'S IT!" he called out, pointing at the monitor. "That's the story right there. That's the end of the story."

Somebody asked whether there were control slices—brain slices from rats that had not gone through the experiment—to examine for comparison purposes. One of the students shouted, "Controls are for wimps!"

This tickled Lynch. "Controls?" he shouted. "Who needs controls?"

Lynch wondered aloud if the slides weren't being kept under the microscope for too long; the intense light could literally burn the brain tissues on the slides, rendering them useless. "We're going to look at all of these. We're going to write the paper, then we're going to come back to these, and they're going to be bleached out, and then I'll go get the Uzi and it will be terrible."

Back at the microscope, he followed the path of the labeled spines through to the hippocampus. Fedulov, who was still new to the lab and more than a little uncertain of his status within it, was standing behind Lynch, grinning widely. Lynch murmured,

"Vadim, Vadim, I'm going to make you famous. . . . That's it. That is the first demonstration that LTP is engaged in memory.

"*Is* memory," he emphasized. "It couldn't have been much better. All those years, all those arguments, it's all gone."

After a minute or so of further scanning and examination, he came across some particularly bright, well-delineated dendritic spines. "You see that, boys and girls? Science works!" he shouted. Then more quietly: "It's the most satisfying thing about science—you see the thing. You can't really believe the thing is what you think, but then you see it. It is a huge part of brain function tied up in it. If you don't have that, you don't have cognition."

One day not long afterward, Arvid Carlsson, a Nobel-laureate pharmacologist, visited Lynch at the lab. Carlsson and Lynch had known each other for years, and Lynch had persuaded him to serve as a scientific advisor to Cortex. The meeting was planned as a mere courtesy visit. But when Lynch briefed him on the latest work, Carlsson was enthralled, digging in and asking a score of questions. He was energized and wanted details, down to the calcium channel, explained to him. He had to be hauled out of the room to catch his flight back to Sweden. "To me, it seems so absolutely surprising and convincing," Carlsson said. "It makes so much sense. It seems to be a fundamental discovery."

The approbation of a learned and widely respected old hand like Carlsson was gratifying to Lynch, who had spent so much of his career struggling for recognition and growing bitter in its absence. But to a surprising extent, he had now moved beyond needing it. He was certain that the delineation of LTP the lab had revealed was such a fundamental brain process that affirmation would come. What mattered now was that the science had finally yielded. He had broken the code. He wanted to see everything the code had obscured. Quite simply, he was greedy. He wanted more.

Those days in the lab were uncharacteristically sunny. Lynch at times was absolutely buoyant. He accepted an invitation to appear on a PBS roundtable discussion on the ethics of bio-enhancement. The other guests included prominent ethicists, writers, scientists, and U.S. Supreme Court justice Antonin Scalia. The discussion took place in Washington, D.C., and began early on the morning after a rather too celebratory dinner party welcoming the participants to town. At one point in the discussion the neuroscientist Tim Tully remarked that he didn't really care about the invention of cognitive-enhancement drugs. He looked forward to the day, he said, when you could take a pill to cure the red-wine hangovers afflicting several of the panelists. Scalia said: "Will it work for Scotch?"

CHAPTER ELEVEN

The Kids

THE ENGRAM, SUMMER 2006

For decades an unrelenting problem in memory research had been to determine the location of long-term memory storage. Tim Bliss once observed that while science made great progress understanding the physiology of the brain and the psychology of cognitive behavior, memory storage remained "a great sea in between." "One of the darkest areas of research," Alcino Silva of UCLA called it. "We know nothing about it, literally nothing."

Researchers almost unanimously agreed that the hippocampus played a fundamental role in acquiring new memories, but few thought it was the site of permanent storage. For one thing, it was too small. It simply didn't have the capacity to store a lifetime's worth of memories. Second, people with damage to the hippocampus, like the famous patient H.M., didn't seem able to form new memories but had substantial recall of events that occurred prior to the hippocampal damage. If memories were indeed encoded by the hippocampus, they seemed to migrate to the neocortex for storage. If that somewhat mystic concept were true, who or what moved them?

Because Lynch Lab now had a technique to see actual memory traces, the scientists thought they ought to be able to plot them onto maps of the brain. What they had done so far was really just a demonstration that such a mapping project was feasible. Real maps, real engrams, Lynch thought, would have nearly unimagined explanatory power. "No question, the maps will change everything," he said. "They'll finally stretch the neurobiology into psychological questions."

As work on the maps got under way, the scientists quickly realized how complicated even a simple memory is and the degree to which a single memory trace is widely distributed across brain regions. When a rat learned a new smell, the trace of the learning landed in the olfactory bulb, then in the cortex, the hippocampus, and the amygdala, all areas previously implicated in memory. The same event showed up all over the brain. In a single stroke, the images seemed to yield a realistic hypothesis for long-term storage. The memory wasn't moved from the hippocampus; rather, it was encoded simultaneously in the hippocampus and in the cortex. Presumably a signal could later be sent from the hippocampus to keep or discard a particular memory. Lynch thought the hippocampus itself retained a sort of index to the memories stored elsewhere, functioning like a card catalog in a library.

Danielle Simmons and Vadim Fedulov, laboring to get the mapping project up and running, proved an imperfect match. Simmons was very much the organized, efficient, and ever-prepared professional; she had spent much of her time in the lab working on Lynch's corporate projects, where erratic grad students weren't welcome. Fedulov was very much the erratic grad student. Bright, inquisitive, inventive? Beyond question. But there was a reason he had been on his way out of academia before Lynch threw him a lifeline. He was unpredictable at best, and stubborn. He and Simmons regularly butted heads, and progress on the mapping was painfully slow. A couple of times, in fact, Lynch came close to firing Fedulov, and once actually did but then relented. As erratic as Fedulov could be (which was plenty), he had the gift that all successful neuroscientists need: the ability to stay at something for a very long time. The problem was getting him locked in.

Whatever complaints Simmons and Fedulov had about each other, however, the main reason for the lack of progress was the phalloidin method itself. Although Lynch was reluctant to credit criticism of it, in truth it was a pain to work with. It sometimes produced spectacular results. Kramar's experiments, after the long nightmare she had been forced to endure en route to her results, yielded truly amazing images. To look at them was to be astonished. But the method proved to be inconsistent, time-consuming, and difficult to execute. In retrospect, her difficulties should have been seen as a warning. If a scientist as punctilious as she has problems making a method work, others are bound to struggle. That the method was ill favored outside the lab was just another problem. As the journal reviewer for Kramar's original paper had put it, the results that were produced using the method "were simply not credible" to some scientists.

A sort of catch-22 was at work. Lynch had given a few talks in which he described the method, and other scientists had come to the lab to learn about it, but its details had not yet been widely distributed. Until Lynch published the details, few other labs could use the method and confirm that it did indeed work. But the fact that no one else was using the method made publishing it problematic, because it contradicted a belief that many neuroscientists held: that phalloidin could not penetrate through a neuron's cell membrane into the cell interior. The basis for this belief was obscure. A single paper had once been published asserting it, and it had somehow become dogma. Although Lynch Lab's experiments seemed to be prima facie evidence to the contrary, the idea that it was somehow impossible persisted. Until something happened to override the belief, Lynch was in a bind.

Kramar, before she left the lab, had suggested to Lynch that maybe they shouldn't be bucking the conventional wisdom. Maybe the critics were right, she said, and some fundamental flaw in the technique had escaped the lab's notice. Maybe the results were artifactual. She told Lynch he might be endangering the careers of the younger members of his team. If the critics turned out to be right, a promising young scientist like Rex would be branded with the failure forever. And in fact, Lynch could be wrong, and what they were doing could fail to revolutionize the world of neuroscience. It might do nothing more than illuminate another blind alley.

Lynch knew this, worried about it almost all the time, and did not take the criticism kindly. When did he ever? Being told to toe the line was not something he ever enjoyed, let alone heeded. When Kramar later told him she was considering taking another job, he encouraged her to go. She was crushed. He resented the imposition of what he viewed as her womanly and wrongheaded emotion into the lab. Of course he cared about Rex's career. He loved the guy. Everybody did. Earlier Rex's car had broken down and somebody stole his backup transport, a bicycle, leaving him with a several-mile walk to and from the lab, which he often completed after midnight; Lynch gave him the old Mustang, which had become a kind of community transit device shared within the lab. But how could he babysit Rex's future? He barely attended to his own. "It's a kid, right? Drop one off a building, and they bounce," he said.

Rex had an "aw, shucks" quality that was as endearing as it was misleading. His apparent softness was mostly affect. He was intense and focused, possessing a rare array of abilities. The neuroscience world was moving to computer-assisted, or controlled, experimentation, and Rex's programming background gave him a huge advantage. So did his ambition. He wanted to do everything. "The kid's like cancer," Lynch said. "One of these days he's gonna come in here and say, 'Sorry, but you'll have to go. I really need this office.'" In lab meetings, if Lynch or Gall suggested a new point of investigation, or a different way to pursue an old one, Rex volunteered to do it. If, after he had taken on more work, yet another avenue of inquiry was proposed, he volunteered to do that one too.

It was clearly crazy, and not sustainable, but it was also in some ways necessary. Lynch, through his disputes with the university—and theirs with him—had backed himself into a corner. The lab had shrunk too much to handle the current onslaught of science. Fate is nothing if not cruel, and the scope of Lynch's science was exploding just as this enforced shrinkage of his research staff was occurring.

Lynch had to some extent believed his own frequent predictions that one day soon—tomorrow, next week, certainly within a month or two—he would solve every outstanding issue to everyone's satisfaction. All the tribes would come to the same campfire, and he could declare victory and go home. (Although not even Lynch believed he would actually go home, not, at least, in the sense of quitting the work; I always thought what he had in mind was something closer to a graceful acceptance of universal acclaim and a pivot to some more abstract, less obviously solvable challenge—seeking the basis of human consciousness, maybe, or the origin of thought.) That this hadn't happened yet, and that Lynch Lab was by and large empty, was not only constraining but somewhat embarrassing. But for the time being, the most obvious result of Lynch's fight with the university was a workload that, if unaltered, would kill Rex before he ever uttered a word of complaint. They'd find him one morning, expired, wearing his cleanest dirty shirt, buried beneath a mound of very nice data. Lynch, of course, had refused Kramar's suggestions on the phalloidin method and soldiered on. Or rather, he'd ordered Simmons to soldier on.

Whatever the world beyond the lab thought of the phalloidin method, Simmons was growing exasperated with it inside. "Phalloidin applied in vivo was transiently visible, and we didn't know why," Simmons said. The stain worked great upon initial application; then, in experiment after experiment, it inexplicably disappeared. Obviously, you couldn't make maps with markers that vanished. Imagine a color-coded map of the United States that attempted to portray, say, age distribution by state, but that had no state borders. The permanence of the markings was an absolute requirement for the construction of the memory maps.

SKIRTS, SUMMER 2006

The phalloidin difficulties were a potentially fatal blow for the mapping project. The stain worked fine for the far briefer amount of time necessary for Kramar's initial work, confirming the structural transformation of the dendritic spine. But the mapping would involve looking at huge swaths of brain tissue, an immensely time-consuming task. If you relied on the method for this work, you might easily miss entire areas where LTP had occurred but where its visible signal had disappeared before you arrived to look.

The phalloidin stain was not intrinsically important; it was merely a marker for the presence of the thing the phalloidin bound to—the polymerized actin. It was possible—indeed, likely—given the number of different proteins involved in LTP, that markers for others could be identified. In some crude sense, much of neurobiology is little more than a search for such bio-markers. Scientists are engaged in a long struggle to see through the darkness. Since they cannot investigate things directly, that is, they can't see them, finding markers that they can see is paramount.

Remember that LTP, although it occurs at what seems like lightning speed, has hundreds of constituent parts, each performing some action necessary to the overall process. LTP is, in effect, not a single event but a process involving long cascades of many events occurring serially within thousands of different neurons at once, so quickly as to seem simultaneous. Lynch focused on actin because it was near the end of the chain and altered its form during the LTP process. Conveniently, the phalloidin marker bound to the actin after it changed form, meaning it "marked" whether LTP had occurred or not.

For the sake of discussion, let's say that LTP involves twenty-six discrete steps. That greatly understates the complexity of the process, but for purposes of illustration it will work. Let's name the steps A, B, C, and so on, through to Z. Step A is sensing some event in the real world. Actin polymerization is step V, toward the end of the process of encoding that real-world event in memory, long after the original sensory experience has been converted to an electrical signal and passed down to the hippocampus. That is why polymerization is so valuable as a marker. Once polymerization occurs, LTP is nearly complete.

Many other proteins are altered during the LTP process. Could an even later protein, one engaged at step X or Y, be identified and marked?

While Simmons and Fedulov soldiered on, trying to make the phalloidin method more consistent, the job of searching for a new marker was given to Lulu Chen, a brand-new grad student in Chris Gall's lab. The assignment's primary intent was to educate Chen in some basic experimental procedures, things as elementary as learning how to use the newer microscopes that were then being incorporated into the lab by the technologically minded Rex. The project was somewhat of a shot in the dark.

Chen had arrived in Gall's lab in July 2006 via a roundabout route. She was born in Taiwan, and her family had come to California when her older sister enrolled in art school here. Her mother couldn't bear to have her oldest child that far from home, so asked her husband, a surgeon, to retire, then moved the entire family to the San Gabriel Valley in suburban Los Angeles. Chen spoke no English, but her high school, located in the center of one of southern California's many immigrant-rich locales, was so heavily Chinese she seldom needed to. Her language skills became a more bracing problem when she enrolled in college at

Cal State, Long Beach. She majored in chemistry mainly to avoid speaking English.

"My friends were writing research papers on Shakespeare and I was learning to spell *table*," she said. She nonetheless had a stellar undergraduate career, but put her schooling aside for several years after graduation to help in her mother's business. One of her mentors at Cal State had attended Irvine, so when she was ready to go to graduate school, she applied there and to UCLA. Accepted at both, she feared she'd party too much in Westwood and chose Irvine. She felt keenly unprepared.

"I have no experience in biology. I don't even know how to use a pipette," she said, "but I liked the idea of being in a biology lab. You could wear skirts, have nail polish. Nail polish wouldn't last five minutes in a chemistry lab. The first day, when I walk in, she [Gall] says, 'Are you okay with animal work?'

"I think, 'What's that mean?'

"I say, 'Of course.'"

They then entered the lab, where she was introduced to Rex, who, inside of the first five minutes Chen had ever spent in a biology lab, guillotined the head off a rat, cracked open its skull, and sliced out the hippocampus. Blood squirted. The headless body twitched in the sanitary waste can. Chen twitched too, "jumping all over the place inside, trying to appear calm outside," she said.

Once over the shock, she took to the work immediately, learning the basic tools of neurobiology. Rex gave her initial training on a confocal microscope, which uses lasers to focus light at any desired depth within fluorescent-stained tissue, yielding virtual 3D images. Rex had just started using it himself and wasn't expert with it. "He knew how to turn it on," Chen said.

The microscope wasn't actually even in the Gall Lab. Confocals were expensive, costing more than $100,000, and neither Lynch nor Gall had budgeted for one out of their grants, so the researchers had to rent time on another lab's apparatus in the basement of Gillespie Hall, where Gall's lab was located.

It is impossible to overestimate the importance, for grad students, of mastering basic practices. Even the simplest experiments have so many variables that not to control the things that need to be controlled made any results nearly useless. One reason neurobiology labs are so quiet is that researchers concentrate intently on the most mundane tasks, trying to eliminate variability wherever they can. First and most important, the researchers are dealing most often with living brain tissue. The health and history of the brain is itself variable. Individuals range greatly in their ability to slice and mount the tissue. The chemical reagents used in experiments are commercially produced, and suppliers sometimes, without notice, change formulas when existing stocks are exhausted. Times and temperatures have to be exact.

Chen was nearly overwhelmed initially and felt certain she would never master the craft. She had a hard time learning the staining techniques but persisted. When she found out she could get time on the confocal microscope for half price at night, wanting to give herself as many opportunities as she could, she started renting the microscope for the entire night. When sleep was absolutely unavoidable, she slept for a couple of hours at a time in her Toyota sedan in the parking lot outside. Inside, she played with the confocal, trying different protocols, just to see what happened, doing science in its oldest sense—exploring. She begged lab mates for any extra brain tissue they weren't using just so she could continue her practicing.

"If I go home, I toss and turn, I can't sleep. I think, 'I should be in the lab.' I'm trying to catch up. That's how I feel," she said. So she would get up, get dressed—in her skirts—and go back to the lab. The training period lasted several months.

Because the phalloidin project was stalled, the search for a new marker took on more importance. If Simmons truly couldn't make the phalloidin method simpler and more reliable, it was hard to see how they could proceed. Some sort of marker was essential. Lynch didn't much care what it was, so long as he had one that worked. Frustrated by the problems and the resulting delays, he turned his attention to ways in which the lab's new techniques and knowledge could be applied directly. He initiated several disease-specific investigations, starting separate projects on Huntington's disease (HD) and Fragile X mental retardation, some of which seemed promising but all of which were in their early stages.

"HD will become a test bed for fixing memory and cognition," Lynch predicted.

> Otherwise-intact young adults with no symptoms but serious memory problems—we know that LTP is busted and BDNF fixes it. Much like the C-Rex middle-aged result [in which application of BDNF had erased cognitive deficits]. And assuming his impression is right, it fixes it by restoring actin polymerization to the spines. There's a great animal model, so we can do the in vivo thing. Isolating where the disease first acts will reveal a ton. The lovely part for me is that it shows the power of what we got over the past year.

The work on Fragile X revealed some similarities between it and Huntington's. "It turns out that there are many ways to foul up the integrin-actin-shape-change-LTP process," Lynch said. "And we do, in fact, know how to override, force our way through, the block."

EMINENT DOMAIN, SUMMER 2006

That summer of 2006, progress came to a halt. "It's hard to explain this lull we're in," Lynch said. "I'm feeling more and more like I'm stuck in some cheesy version of *Moby-Dick*. Remember the part where they lose the wind and drift aimlessly? Maybe I better nail a doubloon to the mast."

It was an apt metaphor. In the category of obsessive pursuits—men flailing against nature, losing body parts and sanity in the process—Captain Ahab had nothing on Lynch. Ahab spent two voyages, at most a matter of months, hunting his fabled white whale; Lynch had invested three decades and counting in search of his. He was so close now, he felt he could nearly touch the thing, yet it remained hidden and beyond reach.

Doubloons, it so happened, weren't the answer. Phosphate groups were. One of the most common actions individual proteins undergo in mammalian biology is a process called phosphorylation. Biochemically, that means a small group of atoms called a phosphate group is added to a protein. Twenty percent of the energy produced by the body is used by the brain, and much of this is used to continuously manufacture the phosphate groups, combinations of phosphorous and oxygen atoms, ensuring their availability whenever needed. Attaching a phosphate group to a molecule is a humdrum biological occurrence—it happened dozens of times while you read that last sentence—but the local effect of phosphorylation is often dramatic, the equivalent of an on-off switch for the protein. In LTP, phosphorylations of several proteins are key steps in the process.

A friend of Gall's, upon reading a draft of the original phalloidin paper, had raised a question about the phalloidin labeling, wondering if it was at all related to cofilin, a protein that was known to bind to actin. Gall didn't know but thought the idea was worth following up. Even before the difficulties with the phalloidin method were clear, Gall had begun urging an investigation into the viability of using fluorescent markers for cofilin and another late-acting protein, PAK (P21-activated kinase), in place of phalloidin. The two were among the first candidates for a late-stage marker that Gall asked Chen to investigate.

Cofilin's normal role is to stop actin from polymerizing, that is, to keep it from reassembling when it is in its broken-down state. During LTP, cofilin is phosphorylated. This effectively turns cofilin off and thus permits polymerization to go forward. Imagine an assembly line that is constantly manufacturing bits of actin. Cofilin sits at the end of the line, and every time a piece of actin rolls off it, cofilin whacks it with a hammer, preventing it from being assembled into the cytoskeleton. After cofilin is phosphorylated, it loses the ability to attack the actin, allowing assembly to go forward. This is yet one more example of what a bizarre mess human biology is. Memory encoding happens because something is turned off?

Chen was assigned the task of determining whether cofilin could be marked. This irritated Rex, who felt a proprietary ownership of almost every new undertaking in the lab. "I was a little miffed," he said. "I wanted it. Obviously, I want everything. It was a struggle in the beginning to let somebody else do it."

Chen eventually found that both cofilin and PAK could be fluorescently tagged. Then it was a matter of perfecting methods to do it. Finally, in early August, after weeks of working out her own protocols, she had a tissue sample in which the fluorescent staining seemed to have worked. Uncertain, she asked Rex to check her work, to see if she had made mistakes. "I think I've got one that's okay," she told him as he sat down at the microscope for a look.

He was shocked. The staining was perfect.

"Okay? You think this is okay?" Chen pleaded.

"Okay? Okay? Oh my god, this is awesome!" Rex yelled. The next day Gall and Lynch were summoned for a look. Like Rex, they were startled. The markers were perfect. Not only were they completely unambiguous, they were also limited to the dendritic spines where polymerization had occurred. The phalloidin method stained actin not just in the spines but also farther down the dendritic tree. At the very least staining more of the dendrite created visual noise in the images. Restricting the staining to the spines made the resulting images that much more discrete, readable, and powerful. Moreover, the stained proteins were located right at the tips of the spines, precisely at the point where synapses form. It was exactly the kind of marker they needed.

Lynch immediately initiated experiments to determine how intimately involved in LTP the two molecules were. Chen and Rex quickly demonstrated that blocking cofilin or PAK stops polymerization, that is, blocks LTP. Even though it had produced stunning images, Lynch stopped all work on the phalloidin project, which not that long before seemed en route to producing—for the first time in human history—detailed and definitive maps of where memories are made in the brain. Lynch thought the new markers would allow him to see deeper into the LTP process.

The markers were easier to use and produced vivid, easily replicable results. And because two markers were being used rather than one, the method provided a means to test the experiments against one another. The confocal could image individual spine heads, a resolution the fluorescent microscopes being used in the phalloidin experiments could not match. This allowed Lynch to address fundamental questions he had first posed decades before: Would the spine heads be larger? If they were, would the extra room allow more AMPA receptor molecules to come to the surface of the spine?

Remarkably, Chen and Rex answered both questions affirmatively within a week.

"Rex and Lulu are absolutely out of their minds," Lynch said.

The method worked perfectly. It's fucking unbelievable. After twenty-six fucking years, after Kevin Lee and I did that EM thing, after we published it in the 1984 paper. It's not just that we got the mechanism, it's that it is almost to the T what I said it was going to be in 1984. This is not just LTP.

> It goes all the way down. . . . We may be the first human beings to sit down and actually stare at the engram.

I asked Lynch if that was it then, if he believed that success in these experiments had proven his LTP hypothesis correct. Well, he said, maybe, maybe not. Then he repeated something he had told me when I first came to the lab the year before:

> Belief is a tricky business. It's funny. No matter how much I know, and knew, it to be the case, I've never been quite able to just believe it and go on. There's another factor: it seems implausible to me that we could have picked out the mechanism for LTP-memory almost from first principles and actually got it right. Takes a lot of stuff to overcome the simple weirdness of it all.

While declaring almost daily that he was about to quit the whole enterprise, Lynch couldn't help himself. Using the new biological markers, the researchers examined numerous disease conditions for LTP deficiencies. The experiments indicated that Huntington's, Parkinson's, mental retardation, and, out of left field, menopause all gave evidence of LTP deficiencies well before any physical symptoms appeared. More astonishingly, the lab revived the Chris Rex protocols in which he had used ampakines to restore loss of cognitive function in middle-aged lab rats and did the same for Huntington's and mental retardation. That is, they cured the rats.

Lynch decided to move directly to behavioral studies without further demonstration of the technique. He commandeered rats that had been trained by Linda Palmer, the philosophy professor, who was trying to determine whether there were patterns of brain activity that correlate with Immanuel Kant's *Critique of Judgment*.

Palmer objected: "What are you doing to my rats?"

"It's martial law," Lynch said. "I've taken over. We're killing them. An act of eminent domain."

Palmer's rats had been trained in a learning task that took advantage of their—and almost all mammals'—inclination to explore novel surroundings. The rats were put in a new, so-called enriched environment, which basically meant they were moved from their sterile home cages and put in a square box that had objects and walls within it. They were allowed to roam throughout, learning the lay of the land without any sort of prompting or cues from the researchers. Even such unsupervised training, as it was known, presumably would have the same sort of effect on neurons that artificially induced LTP had. That is, the rats would learn, and the learning would be encoded in LTP-induced neural networks.

With the rats already trained by Palmer, Lynch anticipated getting proof of learning-induced LTP-type changes within days, a week at most. Ahab would have known better. First, the confocal microscope broke. Rex found another, underused scope across campus, so they had to hustle back and forth with their tissue slides every day, or night. Between the broken scope and other delays, summer passed with the experiments still undone. Lynch was so irate that he considered (but ultimately resisted) violating what he called "the first rule of white males—never, never spend your own money" and buying a microscope out of his own pocket.

Then came another intrusion of the ordinary. "There's this thing called Labor Day, and then there's this thing called students, who think it means road trip," he complained. "Sweet Jesus, but the system is nuts."

After that minor outbreak of students acting like students (in non-Lynchian terms, known as being human), the doldrums were vanquished. Over the next months the team found it could readily identify any individual spine that had undergone LTP.

When they measured the marked spines, they found that they had in fact subtly changed shape, presumably as a result of changes to the actin cytoskeleton beneath them.

The fluorescent microscope images in Kramar's phalloidin polymerization studies had been striking. She used a stain that caused the dendrites where LTP had occurred to fluoresce a brilliant red against the pitch-black background of the rest of the tissue. The results were gorgeous, the long thin lines of the dendrites snaking across the darkness, the nubs of individual spines glowing like stars in the night sky. One oddity was immediately obvious, however. There were an awful lot of things glowing. Theoretically, any one individual memory would consist of a network containing a very, very small percentage of the available neurons and, even within a single neuron, very small percentages of the tens of thousands of available synapses. Kramar's images contained what appeared to be much more staining than that. In some cases an entire dendritic branch was glowing. This same amount of staining showed up in the rats Fedulov had run through the olfactory learning tasks. If that much neural material was polymerized during a single episode of learning, a rat would run out of neurons very quickly. Lynch recognized this as a problem at the time but stashed it in the Worry About It Later file.

The accidental wisdom of letting difficult things sit for a while—that is, ignoring them and hoping they go away—was immediately apparent in the new studies done by Rex and Chen. The number of spines marked using the new double-labeling technique was quite small, less than 1 percent of the spines in any particular region. And there was very little marking whatsoever beyond the spine. The dendritic branches were barely marked at all. The results were unnervingly close to what one might hypothesize.

"The way those numbers work out, it is so close to the expected result that it's hard not to give in and believe," Lynch said. "Fortunately, large numbers [of experimental results] are coming through, and it will make it or not, but everyone now has tasted it, and it is no longer an abstraction. The game really is afoot."

The notion that the end of LTP was approaching made Lynch wistful, even a touch melancholic. Not that everything had gone according to plan: ironically, the new method, which had been intended to serve the engram-mapping project, stopped the mapping dead in its tracks. The new markers had revealed too much new biology to ignore. They brought whole new vistas into view.

For one thing, the new method appeared to show that a very small number of spines was labeled before LTP, or learning, had occurred. This was probably impossible, certainly weird. If the labeling was due to LTP and if LTP was in fact the biological underpinning of learning and memory, how on earth could you have labeling without LTP? In other words, how could you have the biological marker of memory encoding without memories having been encoded? This seemed spooky to everyone who looked at it and suggested some error had been made along the way. But further investigation indicated that a small set of spines was, in fact, always teetering on the brink of potentiation. Natural brain rhythms seemed to create conditions in which they could be easily pushed over the edge.

"This is starting to look quantum and probabilistic," Lynch said.

Spines are on a threshold where they pop in and out of the potentiated state. Theta bursts easily shove the stimulated guys over the top, which makes consolidation machinery set in motion by theta bursts the real secret to the whole thing. The system in its complexity has an equilibrium point—stay here or go there. Like a polity, it's balanced, but barely. The real rate limiting condition is stabilization, anchoring the thing in the potentiated state.

Try as they might, the scientists couldn't get rid of the effect. It seemed to be not an artifact of the experiment, but a real condition in the real world, made apparent for the first time by the new marking protocols. Chen and Rex, while trying to get Lynch off their backs, had unveiled something no one—literally no one—had ever even guessed at. The result seemed to appear out of nowhere, with no hypothetical basis. One reason probably had to do with the way the entire enterprise of LTP research had evolved. In order to understand how and when LTP occurred, researchers had focused very narrowly on discrete events within the broader process. They were following classically reductionist logic, trying to find the smallest piece of information with which they could explain the broader phenomenon. Somewhere along the way they had gotten lost down in the details and for the most part ignored the fact that if LTP were the underpinnings of memory, it had to be a more or less continuous process. It wouldn't be memory otherwise. The field, including Lynch, needed to pull back and look at LTP in a broader context.

There was no time now, or apparent method, for testing any of this. The lab was overrun with results generated using the new method. That fall they reliably demonstrated that the re-modeled synapses were about one-third larger, making room for more receptors, as Lynch had predicted decades before. He and his crew were at full sail, destination unknown. "The hoot for me is in the discoveries, and in the suspicion that something is waiting around the corner," Lynch said. "Lose that sense of mystery? Pull the plug. Can't remember ever feeling better about having bet a life on this thing."

One day, in the middle of an excited commentary on the progress Rex and Chen were then making, Lynch paused, shook his head, and laughed. "It's amazing!" he said. "They just show up. When you need them, there they are. You didn't even know you needed them, and there they are."

He was speaking specifically of Chen, but she was merely the latest miracle to land on his doorstep. It went all the way back to the late 1970s lab, when Mike Browning (a cowboy English major in love with Emmylou Harris) and Kevin Lee (the ringer shortstop) appeared out of the mist, unbidden and essential. Two years ago it had been Rex (art major turned virtual reality coder). "One of these days," Lynch said, "I'll make up a list of the shoe salesmen, shortstops, philosophers, guys who crashed their planes, computer freaks, and so on that played critical roles."

Chen had progressed so quickly, it was scary, Lynch said. She "has a deep intuitive understanding of this and the pleasure that goes with it. Not just uncovering all the chemical links, but with each link a growing belief in the whole."

In the lab, Chen's freshness to the material—in other words, her ignorance—became her ally. "I'm the blind experimenter," she said. "I don't even know what I want to see. I think if I do twenty experiments, I'll fail nineteen times. After I've done ten, I think, 'Good, I've failed halfway to success.' "

All that this approach—the embrace of failure—required was infinite patience and energy. She and Rex became a team, each amping the other's intensity. Soon enough you couldn't get either of them out of the lab.

ATLANTA, AUTUMN 2006

Lynch was feeling so spry and optimistic that for the first time in years he agreed to attend the annual Society for Neuroscience (SFN) convention and to speak at a special LTP convocation that would precede it. The convention that year was in Atlanta in October; the LTP meeting was organized as a tribute to Tim

Bliss, who was retiring. Bliss hadn't added much to the science of LTP following his initial discovery work with Terje Lomo, but he had been a gracious and convivial colleague—an avuncular presence in many respects—to everyone in the field. Lynch and Bliss had been longtime friends, and Lynch felt obligated to attend the meeting. He was also following Gall's long-standing advice to reengage the field; and above all, he had a story he wanted to tell.

Some scientists can, and do, spend as much time attending conferences as doing science. The annual SFN conventions—referred to within the field, like Madonna or Elvis, by the single word *Neuroscience*, as in, "We were at Neuroscience"—are huge, scientifically rich, and socially vibrant events, among the largest scientific meetings held anywhere. In many years attendance tops thirty thousand, and literally hundreds of symposia are conducted, a measure of the breadth of the science the field seeks to cover and, no less important, the networks one needs to build and maintain in order to navigate complicated terrain. These social aspects of the undertaking cannot be overestimated. Grad students finally get a few guilt-free days off. Fresh graduates, with résumés and journal reprints in hand, scour the place plotting postdoc appointments. Alliances are formed or forgotten. Information is exchanged. And the meetings, at least as experienced within Lynch's circle, are tremendous parties. Gone were the days when an army of protégés massed to greet Lynch's arrival, but he still gathered a pretty good-sized and boisterous crowd. He was greeted warmly in Atlanta. "Great to see you back, great to see you," said one scientist after another, clasping Lynch by the arm and squeezing with what seemed genuine affection.

Throughout the meetings old friends and unknown opponents sought out Lynch for intense, sometimes needy, sometimes nervous hallway conversations. At night he was surrounded in the convention hotel bar; it was as if they had reserved a seat, waiting for his return. Single-malt Scotches rained down from on high.

In his talk at the LTP symposium, Lynch generously laid the blame for all the wasted careers represented by those present on "the great terrible mess that Dr. Bliss sent out into the world." Lynch parceled out a few of the details he and his colleagues had added to the LTP story, but remained somewhat oblique about the lab's most recent advances. He didn't use the word *engram*, which by then had acquired the musty smell of failure, but nonetheless hinted that his lab might have at long last found a means to map memories. Peter Seeburg, a German scientist and longtime friend, challenged Lynch on the mapping, wondering how it was even conceivable that one could find a single memory among many thousands or millions.

Lynch, in his best autodidactic mode, replied that Seeburg was probably right, unless the test animals were rodent Kaspar Hausers, a reference understood quite possibly only by Lynch and Seeburg, a German. Hauser was a German boy who had been locked in a basement until a teenager, whereupon he turned up unknown and unknowing on the streets of Nuremberg. The Lynch Lab rats were kept in cages, undernourished neurologically before the experiment. The researchers were writing on the blank slate of the rats' lack of experience, he said.

He showed slides of Kramar's striking phalloidin polymerization studies but didn't even mention the advances Chen and Rex had since made with cofilin and PAK. "We don't do complicated methods out in Irvine," he said. "We're simple people."

Several scientists were dubious. The news about the phalloidin method had been seeping out for months, but some guessed there was something more. "You've got a new marker, haven't you?" they asked. Lynch tried to be coy but as usual couldn't pull it off. He'd grin one of his lopsided grins and shrug. Such moments revealed Lynch, charmingly, for the naïf he in many ways was. He was the damnedest sort of intellectual sophisticate, able at a moment's notice to muster powerful, nuanced arguments on the most abstruse philosophical points, to discuss with forbidding intellectual force a frightening range of subjects, yet utterly at a loss to bluff his way past the least revelation of what he might be fibbing about. He could dissect the arc of thirty years of fiction from Pynchon, DeLillo, and Roth, yet hadn't a clue what wine to order with dinner. He was in many ways still the awkward, ill-fitting kid from Wilmington; a kid, to be sure, with a really, really good brain, but a kid nonetheless.

The big news of the meeting was a frontal attack on Lynch's hypothesis announced by a little-known scientist, Todd Sacktor, from the State University of New York Downstate Medical Center in New York City, not heretofore known as a neuroscience hot spot. Sacktor presented evidence that he had found an enzyme, called PKM zeta, that was all by itself largely responsible for maintenance of long-term memories. If you disabled the enzyme hours or even days after a memory was formed, the memory disappeared, he said.

This seemed rather unlikely to a lot of people. One dismissed it as "hand-waving," a reference to a magician's hocus-pocus onstage and a polite way of calling someone else's results farfetched. Nobody was more invested in a model of memory that would make such a discovery impossible than Lynch. Sacktor had approached Lynch before he presented his results and did so again afterward. He was almost apologetic. Lynch, though, was unaccountably thrilled. He saw something of himself in Sacktor, an outsider challenging the powers that be. That didn't mean he accepted Sacktor's results.

"You understand this is radical new biology?" he asked Sacktor.

"Reluctantly, but yes," Sacktor replied.

Later that day Lynch and a few people from his lab sneaked

out of the convention to a bar to watch a baseball play-off game. During the game the discussion turned to the location patterns of major-league pitchers. These patterns hadn't changed in decades, perhaps centuries. Pitchers typically start by trying to throw a fastball—a relatively straight pitch—for a strike, then maybe follow that with another fastball before switching to pitches that are slower but move in various directions, usually away from the hitter, according to what sort of spin the pitcher imparts to the ball by changing his grip, arm angle, or release. In addition to changing spins and speeds, pitchers also move the ball in and out relative to the batter, pitching inside, then out. Everybody knew this. After a Detroit Tiger pitcher threw a pitch high and inside to an Oakland A batter, the television announcer broadcasting the game said the pitcher's next pitch probably would be a curveball low and away. It was an unexceptional prediction. Why, then, if the announcer in the broadcast booth in Oakland knew it and everybody in the bar in Atlanta knew it and even Uncle Ed in Bangor knew it, why didn't the batter know it? It seemed a real-world example of Lynch's LTP rules. The batter intellectually knew everything that others knew and almost certainly more, but the high-and-tight fastball had concentrated his attention, causing the LTP machinery to kick in and the path that fastball had taken up near his head to be filed away. When the next pitch—it was, as predicted, a breaking ball that started on the same path as the prior pitch, but curved dramatically away at the end—came, the batter flinched involuntarily, then swung weakly and missed.

He couldn't help himself; the automatic categorization rules of LTP filed that second pitch in the same category as the first. No matter what the hitter knew, his brain knew better. The brain was wrong, of course, and caused him to swing and miss.

The hitter who is able to erase the memory of that prior pitch before the next one comes is the one who will be able to assess it objectively, to negate the categorization machinery, to exercise judgment. It's easy to see how this ability can apply in other circumstances. It can be the activity that underlies someone's ability to "be in the moment," to experience events as they occur and not conflate them with expectations drawn from prior events. It doesn't have to be baseball players. It can be actors or politicians or someone driving down the street. In normal circumstances, developing a catalog of expectations can be a very good thing. It kept our ancestors from walking past the glen where the saber-toothed tigers lay; it keeps most of us from needlessly antagonizing our bosses. Under some circumstances, however, experience is not the best teacher but the worst.

Lynch agreed with the general conclusion but seemed preoccupied: not with the game, which was a desultory affair. After a while he said, "It's impossible, of course, and it scares the hell out of me."

He wasn't talking about baseball. He was talking about Todd Sacktor: "Todd's a serious guy. He understands the constraints."

Lynch had been meticulously gathering evidence for decades to support the hypothesis that a structural reorganization of neurons undergirds the encoding of long-term memories. Now along comes a guy with an experimental result, completely out of the blue, that would undermine everything Lynch had done. Sacktor's findings were a perfect illustration of what Lynch had often said—belief is a tricky business, and you have to be excessively careful. You have to have ideas and pursue them with vigor, but you also have to regard all your assumptions as rebuttable. Everything you know is always at risk. If you are truly doing science, you can get your hat handed to you at any moment.

He elaborated later:

Todd claims to have discovered the substrate of long-lasting memory, a claim that depends little if at all on LTP. He is free to borrow what he likes from the field. For example, he uses my actin polymerization results—indeed, downloads the model to explain memory for first one to two hours—and throws the rest of it away. Like me, Todd could replace LTP. Reductionism works. No, the fascinating point is that the mechanism is inherently implausible. It's radical biology, and the problems pile up quickly, maybe more quickly than Todd realizes.

Lynch said he would devise experiments to test Sacktor's findings as soon as he returned to Irvine, which he did. He handed the task off to Eni Kramar, who had resigned from the university but continued to come in on weekends to work on a few pet projects. Sacktor's discovery, like so many others in neuroscience, was based not on actual observation but on an inference. That is, he had used a chemical to block the action of his target, the PKM zeta enzyme. After he did so, he determined that his test animals were incapable of performing tasks they had previously mastered. He then inferred that blocking the enzyme blocked the memory and that the enzyme therefore was crucial to long-term memory.

Sacktor wasn't by training a physiologist and seemed not to appreciate the complexity and varied interactions that occur within a hippocampal slice. Kramar was not the person you would want examining your unusual results. If there was a flaw in your work, she would find it. She would bend over backward to be fair, but she would seize the flaw and beat you to submission with it. Your theory would be dead before you knew it was under attack. What Kramar found was that the chemical Sacktor used to block the action of the enzyme he was interested in blocked almost everything that might happen along the signaling pathway he was examining. Kramar tried as best she could to reproduce Sacktor's result without killing other activity in her brain slices—and couldn't do it.

Sacktor's result, indeed, seemed to be a bit of hand-waving.

When you take a step back, however, almost all neuroscience results contain some greater or lesser element of hand-waving. Our actual knowledge of what is going on within the brain when memories are made is shocking in its absence. The lack of broad theory in which to fit the individual bits and pieces that different scientists were describing is striking.

By some counts more than one thousand different kinds of proteins are present at a single synapse. There were during the three-day LTP conference fifty thirty-minute talks, almost all of them devoted to discussion of different, particular molecules. Little was offered in the way of a theory as to how the brain actually works or how memory is encoded. The five days of the broader neuroscience meeting that followed were much the same. And almost every talk contained at its core some bit of hand-waving, some magic that inexplicably accounted for whatever was being examined.

An essential thing about magic is that once revealed, it isn't very magical. The man in the black suit who makes the apple disappear almost certainly ends up with an apple hidden in his baggy back pocket. Magic is illusion, and the grim facts that make the illusion possible—the special deck of cards, the hidden pocket, the substitute coin—are unforgivingly banal. Lynch's big bet was that the biology of memory is equally banal. In his version of the trick, there were no magic enzymes allowed.

CHAPTER TWELVE

The Failure of Science

DRUGS, JANUARY 2007

In the two years from New Year's Day 2005 to New Year's Day 2007, the Lynch and Gall labs laid out in Cajalian detail a description of LTP, complete with photographic evidence, that overwhelmed anything that had come before it. They now knew and had demonstrated what LTP was, how it happened, its time course, and that it happened not just in the laboratory but in the brain during actual behavior. The scientists were still working to demonstrate the final, consolidating steps that stabilized LTP and made it irreversible, but in some sense that now seemed more like housekeeping than new science.

The lone dark cloud in the Lynch universe was Cortex. After the FDA had ordered a halt to all further ampakine CX717 trials in the spring of 2006, the company waited weeks to get an explanation. When it finally came, it seemed improbable. In the course of examining tissue samples the company had given to the agency, government scientists noticed abnormalities in brain tissues from monkeys Cortex had used to test the toxicity of its drug. In Cortex's tests the monkeys had exhibited no ill effects from having been given the drugs; in fact, the very presence of the drugs wasn't evident from observation. When Cortex autopsied the animals after they had been sacrificed, the brain samples had been unexceptional in every way. Now, however, the FDA claimed there were abnormalities in some of the tissues and wanted to know what had caused them.

Never having seen the effect themselves, Cortex's scientists had no idea where the problem arose. For a time they thought the monkeys might have had some sort of virus before Cortex ever obtained them. Eventually, and after some difficulty, they determined that the abnormalities the FDA discovered were a "postmortem effect"—that is, chemicals used to preserve the brain tissue were apparently to blame. Cortex submitted these results back to the FDA, then confidently awaited notice as to when they could resume the trials. So far as anyone knew, the FDA had never stopped a drug trial because of postmortem effects. The general feeling was that the widely publicized problems with the painkiller Vioxx, which had had to be withdrawn from the market because of serious safety concerns, had brought in a renewed sense of caution at the FDA. In rounds of blame-fixing, the FDA had been heavily criticized for its cozy relationships with the pharmaceutical industry. Much of the criticism was deserved, but the FDA was severely hamstrung in dealing with the issues the Vioxx episode brought to light. The agency had been underfunded for several years and had more than five hundred unfilled positions within its ranks. More important, the agency had never really had the wherewithal to exercise responsibility over drugs once they got to market. Its principal charge had been to oversee testing prior to a drug being approved for sale. After a drug passed those tests, it was for all practical purposes up to its manufacturer to determine whether any health problems were associated with taking the drug.

In any event, FDA decisions could not be appealed. The agency answered mainly to Congress, and Congress was not likely to take up arms on behalf of a drug manufacturer. Cortex went to what it considered extreme lengths to reproduce the effect the FDA had found in a single monkey. They were able to produce a similar result in rats, but only after the rats had been subjected to ampakine dosages up to seventy-five times greater than normal. Obviously, giving any medicine in a dose that high could create problems, but the FDA routinely required drugs to be safe at many multiples of normal dosing. The rationale was that a consumer might inadvertently take a much greater dose than prescribed. It was an example of how the same agency could place what seemed unreasonable restrictions on drug makers while simultaneously being accurately accused of lax oversight.

In late October the FDA notified Cortex that it was lifting the hold on trials but was imposing severe restrictions on the size of dosages that could be used. Citing the reproduction of the anomaly at extreme doses, the agency wanted to see more definitive proof of Cortex's contention as to the source of the problem. Cortex had no choice but to accept the dose limits. It essentially meant the company could not resume the ADHD trials—its most successful to date—because the drug had not been effective in those trials at lower doses. The company could resume Alzheimer's trials but would have to start all over again with drug candidates for other disease indications. This was a gut shot. Nobody had seen it coming. The effect was severe. The day the restriction was announced, Cortex's stock plunged 39 percent.

A pharmaceutical industry analyst wrote: "If the standard of caution being applied now to CX717 were applied to the full range of psychiatric and neurology drugs, it would probably knock out the great majority—as well as aspirin and Tylenol."

In January 2007 Lynch mounted a defense. In the midst of the final stages of the LTP work, the initiation of new work on a variety of disease models, and the long-delayed resuscitation of the mapping program, he threw his lab into the "battle of Cortex . . . many fronts, few troops." He felt, he had said, like Frederick the Great in the Seven Years' War, besieged on all sides by the great powers of Europe. In real life, Frederick had been able to decide his own fate on the battlefield. Lynch wasn't so lucky. The scientists eventually worked out exactly what had caused the problem the FDA had uncovered. They were able to reproduce the exact circumstances and re-create the condition. As they had supposed, the anomaly had had nothing to do with the ampakine. Cortex's upper management actually came over to the university labs to observe a demonstration of the experiments, a very rare event. Sparks and excitement ensued, Lynch said. "C-Rex like a fish in water. Lulu Y. Chen thinking, 'A herd of white males—wow, wonder if I'll ever see this again.'"

The herd, as it happened, was thrilled and rushed the results back to the FDA. Whatever evidence Rex, Chen, and their comrades had been able to muster, the fate of CX717 would be determined in Washington. Lynch was convinced the drug would ultimately be approved. He also thought that its most remarkable aspect had by and large been ignored. "When they give these drugs to rats, rats do things rats can't do," he said. "When they give them to monkeys, monkeys do things monkeys can't do.

The brain, in order to bundle a thought—and everybody agrees with this, too, by the way—has to assemble a transient network of neurons. The neurons are connected at their synapses. So the more complicated the network that you assemble, . . . the greater the probability that some parts of the circuit are going to fail. Now the whole system is massively redundant, so you get away with a lot of that, but nonetheless, reality will kick in at some point. So if you say the farthest two neurons [in a network of neurons that comprise a thought] can't be more than seven or eight synapses apart. . . . Get a drug that will increase the probability of success at these synapses. Now, how big a network can you assemble?

Think about it. The surety of communication between your brain cells with these will be enhanced, okay? Which means that, I think, the size of the network you can assemble will increase. That's where I think things get entertaining. Nothing like this has ever existed.

Here Lynch couldn't stop himself from cackling. If he weren't sitting down, he would at this point be dancing a jig. "It's the end of life as we've known it," he said.

Is that a good thing? I asked.

Lynch stopped laughing and shrugged. "That's the ballad of 'Wernher von Braun,' " he said. "The rockets go up; it's not my job to know where they come down."

Lynch was frustrated less by the FDA's action limiting CX717 doses than by Cortex's apparent inability to move ahead with later incarnations of the ampakines, which in the lab were more powerful yet apparently benign. Lynch had virtually quit experimenting with the older ampakines, while the new ones were being used in investigations of a widening range of indications—mental retardation, Huntington's disease, breathing disorders, old age, menopause.

The disease work was motivated in part by Lynch and Gall's desire to secure NIH funding. Somewhat paradoxically, while one part of the federal government, the FDA, was making it harder and harder to create new drugs, another part, the NIH, was actively pursuing drug creation. Academic science, in the early twenty-first century, had moved ever farther from the old romantic notion of researchers working on problems that attracted their interest. It was now a complicated dance between researchers and funders, as the former forever tried to determine what might lure the interest of the latter. The constant pressure to produce and publish results at least matched the constant stockholder pressure, evident in commercial science, to produce profits. "Your main responsibility as the head of an academic lab is as a procurer of money," said one scientist. "It's a myth that you have academic freedom. You can do science only if somebody will give you money to do science."

The popular push in recent years for special funding to build stem cell programs was a frightening specter to many academic scientists. The voters of California, to cite but one example, had passed an initiative to allocate $3 billion to build and fund stem cell centers. "Man, the boys are backing the Ryder trucks up and filling 'em with cash," Lynch said. "Real research money is drying up so fast it'll soon be memory, so then you dangle stem cell money: water in the desert."

Few scientists had any particular complaints about stem cell research or its potential, but to segregate large amounts of public dollars for a specific sort of research at a time of generally constrained resources was not considered the most rational decision making. Those disinclined or ill prepared to do stem cell work were left to compete for an ever-declining pool of funds. The NIH, conscious of its own need to demonstrate success to its funders in Congress, began emphasizing "translational" research, or academic research that could be translated into medicines or other therapies.

Lynch, after years of being frowned upon for his willingness to mix commerce with science, now found himself in the suddenly popular position of an academic scientist with a long history of commercial involvement. Not that the welcome was full-throated or universal. He still encountered more than his share of adverse reactions. In a review of an NIH grant request, one commenter wrote that Lynch "has been a leader in the LTP field usually ahead of others in conceptual thinking. He has been very productive." The grant proposal, this reviewer said, was solid, well focused, and substantial. The reviewer then concluded by saying he wasn't certain Lynch should get the grant: "It is not clear that the PI [principal investigator] has integrated his work into the wider LTP field or taken advantage of a broader array of tools that are available, for example transgenic animals."

It is hard to imagine how the same reviewer could have made both statements one and two, but it is a good example of the overwhelming normative pressure in science. Step outside the room, and you are liable to get run over by the forces of moderation.

The university gave evidence of the same ambivalence. For years, administrators and colleagues had eyed Lynch's various business entanglements suspiciously; some wondered aloud if they did not present conflicts of interest. Now they heralded his entrepreneurial zeal and honored him at formal dinners. In the spring of 2007, they tried to squeeze more money out of his operation, unilaterally doubling the amount they took out of his grants for overhead. This infuriated Lynch, because every dollar the university took was a dollar unavailable for him to spend on scientists. Furthermore, the overhead costs had been agreed upon before the grants were sought.

Lynch obviously had a vested financial interest in the continued development of ampakine drugs (as did the university, which was coholder of the ampakine patents), but his pursuit of their development was more about pride than money. Having money freed Lynch to do what he wanted, and what he wanted, by god, was to show the bastards. This is not an uncommon motivation among scientists, many of whom, it turns out, are at least as human as Lynch. Their attitudes may derive in part from what they believed about science when they entered it and what they found out about it once in, which was, in short, that it is an uneven meritocracy at best. Not all virtue is rewarded, and some wickedness is. Scientific research is a very human activity, and having overdeveloped intellects doesn't mean that scientists check their emotions at the door.

Tim Tully once told me a story about his childhood in blue-collar Peoria, Illinois. Tully is a tall, strapping fellow who looks as though he might run half marathons at lunchtime. He resembles the actor Bruce Dern and has some of the same manic quality about his eyes. Tully was a gifted swimmer as a boy, but his high school didn't have a swim team. So he competed for a local YMCA team, which, he said, the schoolboys looked down upon. Tully nonetheless won a race in a prestigious statewide championship when he was a junior in high school. The top-ranked swimmer at the distance had missed the meet because of an injury, and Tully's victory was insufficiently appreciated because of that, he said.

"This pissed me off so bad, pissed me off," Tully said.

I arranged to spend the next year doing nothing but get ready for this guy, as the defending champ. The meet the next year is in Peoria, so it's a hometown crowd. The gun goes off, we're gone. I touch the guy out at the wall. I looked up and saw the official signal—my lane. I had won. I got up out of the pool and walked right out of the building. I never swam competitively again. I said, "Take that, you mother-fuckers!" and walked away from it. By that time I had been sick of swimming anyway, but goddammit if they're going to say that about me.

Lynch could not have phrased it better. He wanted the ampakines to succeed because they were his.

PORTALS, SPRING 2007

The Lynch and Gall labs now totaled just a couple of dozen people and lacked the fierce internal rivalries that had so often characterized Lynch's operations. These labs were almost collegial by comparison. Even situations that might have become battle-grounds—the emergence of Chen, for example, as a rival to Rex—instead became scientific group hugs with everybody chipping in to help everybody else.

Most of the work was now being done in Gall Lab, and the change of venue might have been the single biggest reason for the gentler mood. Gall is nearly the polar opposite of Lynch in temperament, an ocean of calm to his mountain of bluster; a major outbreak of emotion from Gall may be to blink her eyes two or three times quickly. She is unflappable. The idea of somebody punching a wall in her lab is unimaginable. She also has none of the enmity with colleagues that Lynch enjoys. To the contrary, she serves on all the department committees, even taking a turn as an officer of the international Society for Neuroscience.

The focus of the research had also shifted subtly. The drive to find markers that could be used to delineate Lynch's hypothetical time course of LTP had created an obsession not with grand design but with infinitesimal details. It was still LTP all day, every day, but the basic principles were no longer in doubt. For the last year the researchers had been drilling farther and farther down into the chemical details. Those details, while sometimes hard to understand, were nonetheless settling nicely into the boxes Lynch had assigned them.

Since the very beginning of his LTP research, Lynch had been trying to standardize the LTP vocabulary. His intent was more than definitional; he wanted to build both a common language and a standard model of the process. Not without incident, he had largely succeeded with both. The most widely used general descriptions of LTP followed Lynch's model—induction, expression, consolidation. He in turn had used the model to organize his investigation, moving through the stages, and the subroutines that arose, in an orderly progression. He was now well into the final pieces of the consolidation stage—in other words, at the very end.

The process had been resolved to a largely accepted standard schematic: theta bursts open channels into the neuron; ion influx activates the disassembly of the cell cytoskeleton; it is followed by reassembly, otherwise known as the actin polymerization machinery; the polymerization leads to a shape-change on the dendritic spine, locked in by the integrins; the shape-change makes room for more AMPA receptors at the synapse. The greater number of receptors strengthens the likelihood of synaptic communication.

Lynch had spent years carving the LTP process into discrete time courses that correspond with the observable facts of memory—that it occurs instantly but can be dislodged and lost if interrupted before it is locked in place. This is the final step Lynch refers to as consolidation. The lab in the past year had dug down deeper into the chemical events that lead to consolidation. Chen eventually found two more proteins that could be marked very near the end of LTP—the protein cortactin and an enzyme awkwardly named calcium-calmodulin sensitive kinase, commonly referred to as CamK-II and spoken of in conversation as cam-kinase two. Both markers are activated by theta bursts and remain at the synapse thirty minutes later, well beyond the time when polymerization occurs. Chen also demonstrated that the initial theta burst, which sets the whole LTP process in motion by releasing neurotransmitters, also releases BDNF from the axon terminal. So not only is the theta rhythm ideal for initiating the process; it is also crucial in providing the materials needed to see it through to the end.

"All these pieces reinforce the initial conclusion that the incredibly brief theta episodes drive long-lasting cytoskeletal reorganization in spines. We will never notice the moment when for the group it transitioned from a scary thing to say, to looks good, to taken for granted. This is very satisfying," Lynch said.

One of the patterns Lynch perceived in the history of science was that a scientific discovery, in order to be meaningful, couldn't be a one-off; it had to connect to a body of knowledge. Otherwise it was meaningless, or at least premature. But once it did connect to that wider body of knowledge, who knew what might happen? Lynch came to regard the invariable surprises as portals into a bigger world. One portal that opened as a result of basic research into LTP was an enhanced ability to examine diseases.

The team had built a stockpile of molecular markers that covered LTP's entire time spectrum. As with Kramar's phalloidin marker and with Lynch's ampakines, they had effectively armed themselves with more tools to probe diseases.

"Right now, we are looking at potential treatments for middle-aged dumbness, mental retardation, Huntington's, and Rett's [a severe breathing disorder that afflicts mainly young girls]. None of this would have made any sense without having linked LTP to basic biology," Lynch said.

> And unbelievably, the new stuff goes directly to the theory of aging, and how longevity is set by another one of those unintended consequences. I argued that dendrites determine life span in mammals, and guessed it was because they must be incredibly stable and therefore not able to replace themselves. This was the deal to get real LTP—spine changes make no sense as memory devices unless the dendrites on which they sit are unchanging. So now we find that the dendrites have very, very low concentrations of the proteins needed to modify the actin cytoskeleton. They must be nonplastic. Next, we'll show that they lost their growth potential at about the time in development that the integrins take over the synapse. Then I'll figure a way to turn 'em back on. Portal is definitely large enough.
>
> The trick is to have a stable marker for potentiated spines. The PAK/cofilin phosphorylation only lasts fifteen minutes or so. Actin polymerization is much longer lasting, but it's a bitch to use with the synapse stains. Still, Rex the wonder boy may have solved this last problem, so we would be able to go out to two hours at least. This could be settled next week. If it breaks the right way, then quantum paper backed up with persistence data are the biggest LTP events in twenty years.

Rex solved the actin problem in mid-January 2007 by using both the new PAK/cofilin markers Chen had found and

Kramar's phalloidin staining method. A type of computer-modulated imaging device that was able to resolve the very slightest signals in tissue picked up even the faint phalloidin signals.

The paper the lab ultimately produced on the Huntington's research was titled "Brain-derived Neurotrophic Factor Restores Synaptic Plasticity in a Mouse Model of Huntington's Disease." This was an astonishing claim. Huntington's is a purely genetic disease. The fatal flaw of the particular gene mutation that produces it was identified long ago, and it has nothing to do with "brain-derived neurotrophic factor," or BDNF, otherwise known to Lynch as Big Deal Neurotrophic Factor. But Rex had found the result the prior year when studying LTP deficits in middle-aged rats. It was too much of a coincidence to be accidental. It suggested that BDNF is even more intimately involved in LTP than anyone had claimed, although by what mechanism was still unknown. As much as Lynch had always mocked the claims for BDNF, the experimental results were rising beyond even the most boisterous claims for its power.

Invariably, after the lab sent a paper to a journal, Lynch was antsy for a period, certain that the universe was conspiring against him once again. The last year's string of publications had diminished the feeling somewhat, but it hadn't disappeared. So it gave him particular pleasure that the Huntington's paper sailed through the review process. He took additional satisfaction from one reviewer's comment. "Remember the outrageous phalloidin method that violated all the laws," Lynch said. "Check out last sentence of the below, just-received review."

The reviewer had written:

Beyond these [minor] issues, the revised manuscript is very much improved and clearly describes an important and exciting set of experiments that significantly advance our understanding of the role of BDNF in cellular models of

learning and memory. The experimental test of the benefits
of wide-field CCD imaging vs. confocal microscopy for the
faint phalloidin staining stands out as an example in meticu-
lousness for others to follow, one that would hopefully con-
tribute to a much needed standardization in the field of
structural plasticity of dendritic spines.

If that were not gratifying enough, the initial reviews on
Chen's quantum spine paper arrived soon thereafter. Just submitting a paper advancing the idea that dendritic spines jump in
and out of potentiated states gave Lynch pause—it was too odd,
too far-fetched. Talking about it in casual conversation, Lynch
would do everything but put air quotes around the phrase *quantum spines*. Even after writing and submitting the paper, he kept
ordering replications of the experiment. When the replications
produced the same results, Rex started doing variations of it.
Simply put, no one really trusted the result. This was odd. For
literally decades Lynch had been criticized for getting out in
front of his data, for falling victim to his own tantalizing stories.
Now here he was with a most fantastic and very nearly complete
story, and he could barely bring himself to tell it.

Then in record time came the reviews: the paper was "a tour
de force," "an extremely interesting study," "quite convincing."
These were not words customarily included in journal reviews,
which prize the particular objection much more than generalized admiration.

Lynch was stunned. "One giant step for mankind," he said.
Then he ordered more experiments. If nobody else was willing
to doubt his results, well, by god, he would. A fundamental difficulty of advanced neuroscience is that the problems scientists
attempt to solve are so difficult and the available experimental
machinery so inept that every result—even the best of them—is
hard to believe.

When he and the lab had finally run enough iterations of the behavior experiment that there was no reasonable way to deny the results, Lynch wrote a paper essentially summarizing thirty years of work. It wasn't stated as an overarching recapitulation, but the title alone made the ambition clear: "Evidence That Long-term Potentiation Occurs Within Individual Hippocampal Synapses During Learning." Trying to determine whether this was in fact true, if LTP was memory, had been the focus of LTP research around the globe since Bliss and Lomo's 1973 discovery.

Lynch wanted to get the paper into print as quickly as possible, and the fastest course available was through *Proceedings of the National Academy of Sciences,* which had a remarkably short turnaround between submission and publication. That journal rejected the paper outright, because the "expert editor who evaluated it concluded that although the work is interesting, it does not have the broad appeal needed for PNAS and is better suited for a more specialized journal."

This was an odd statement: for three decades LTP had probably consumed more careers and money than any other single issue in neuroscience. It addressed a fundamental hypothesis about the human condition—how we learn and remember. Almost ten thousand papers had been written about it. And it wasn't of broad interest?

The rejection was irritating but of little import. Lynch immediately submitted the paper unchanged to the *Journal of Neuroscience,* which accepted it with glowing reviews, the slightest of revisions, and surprising speed. The paper was published in July. The same month the FDA removed the last dosage restriction on CX717, which Cortex took as the final absolution from the agency's prior restrictions. The company applied immediately to the relevant division of the FDA—the Psychiatry Division—to restart clinical trials for ADHD. To do so, Cortex had to go to the end of the line, essentially starting over with the FDA.

AMPAKINES, SUMMER 2007

Cortex had not been alone in its Sisyphean ampakine odyssey. Aside from early successes with antidepressants, which were invented utterly by accident, the entire pharmaceutical industry by and large had failed to produce effective therapies for cognitive diseases. Why was it so hard to make drugs aimed at the brain? Derek Lowe, a pharmaceutical chemist and widely read commentator on the business, wrote:

> It's hard to come up with disease-altering therapies when you don't really understand a single disease in the whole field. . . . We know a lot more than we used to; we know more every year. But we don't know enough to cure anyone yet. Even in the areas where we know more than average, we still don't know enough to step in with therapies that can do what people really want them to do.

More generally, human biology is a singularly messy environment in which to work. "This gets back to a common theme that I stress around here," Lowe wrote.

> Biochemical networks are hideously, inhumanly complex. There's really no everyday analogy that works to describe what they're like, and if you think you really understand them, then you're in the same position as all those financial people who thought they understood their exposure to mortgage-backed security risks. You'll have this enzyme, you see, that phosphorylates another enzyme, which increases its activity. But that product of that second enzyme inhibits another enzyme that acts to activate the first one, and each of

them also interacts with fourteen (or forty-three) others, some of which are only expressed under certain conditions that we don't quite understand, or are localized in the cell in patterns that aren't yet clear, and then someone discovers a completely new enzyme in the middle of the pathway that makes hash out of what we thought we knew about.

To look at but one example, consider Alzheimer's, the most common neurodegenerative disease. Alzheimer's first afflicts the hippocampus. Early symptoms include the incidental episodes of forgetfulness that are often brushed off as "senior moments." The symptoms progress, slowly at first, to more frequent memory disruptions, to broader cognitive problems—confusion, disorganization, disorientation. Eventually, as the disease works its way through ever more areas of the brain, it alters personality and destroys the self, reducing the victim to little more than a warm body greatly in need of care. Death, when it finally arrives, is often welcome.

Thousands of labs across the world—both academic labs like Lynch's and commercial ones—are focused wholly or in part on Alzheimer's. What is most striking about the research is its vast variety. Different scientists blame the disease variously on misfolded proteins, broken neural pathways, misprinted gene maps, or insufficient cellular trash collection. Private industry, from tiny shops like Cortex to the pharmaceutical giants, have laid out plans to fight the disease with all the sophistication and firepower they can muster. They propose treatments as varied as inhaling insulin, eating turmeric, fixing vitamin deficiencies, injecting stem cells, and inventing neuroprotective vaccines—everything, it seems, but altering the phase of the moon.

At conferences, earnest scientists present each potential fix as a likely avenue to pursue. The overall result, however, is a mess. If everything is possible, nothing is likely. In Alzheimer's research, lots of people seem to have quit believing anything is wrong or right or crazy. The simple fact is that after more than a century of research, no one really knows what causes Alzheimer's or how to stop it.

In the United States there are currently five medications approved for treatment of Alzheimer's, one of which causes severe problems so is almost never prescribed. The other four take in an estimated $4 billion a year. They do nothing to stop the disease and have only marginal, often transitory effects on its symptoms. They are on the market because at the moment, other than sympathetic smiles, there is little else to offer people afflicted with the mind-crippling disease. Another fifty-six drugs are in some stage of FDA-regulated clinical trials; few people other than their creators have great hopes for them.

Sometimes not even the creators are optimistic. In 2007 Wyeth, the New Jersey–based pharmaceutical company, announced it had ten candidate Alzheimer's drugs in clinical trials. Ten? From one company? In an industry that typically takes years or decades to produce a single drug candidate and then at costs in the hundreds of millions, Wyeth rolled out ten new compounds? Drug companies have had such a hellish time translating their research into effective neural disease treatments that Wyeth had decided to push everything it had into trials and see what, if anything, worked. Internally, Wyeth called this the "fail faster" approach.

For the person afflicted with the disease, the stakes cannot be higher. Less noted, the stakes for the broader society are just as large. An estimated 6 million Americans have Alzheimer's. That number has lately been growing exponentially, primarily because of medical progress itself. As medical care and therapies improve and people live longer every decade, more and more of them are afflicted with age-related dementias. This will not stop anytime soon, and the cost of treating the disease will go up as well, multiplying as the population continues to age. This year alone Alzheimer's care will cost Medicare an estimated $170 billion.

By 2020 the amount could overtake the defense budget. One analysis has estimated that by 2055 Alzheimer's will cost Medicare more than $1 trillion annually.

While the cost of Alzheimer's soars, federal money spent on research has flattened and is expected to decline in real terms as the competition heightens. The rising costs of treating the disease, coupled with reduced research funding, are foreboding. Andy Grove, the former chairman of Intel Corporation, who has Parkinson's disease, has lamented the lack of a full-scale attack on neurodegenerative disorders:

> We are about to experience an explosion of Alzheimer's disease cases. Population statistics, incident rates, and demographic changes indicate that the incidence of AD is doubling every five years. North America alone is going to have multiple millions of cases in a few more years, and when you look at the economic aspect of this, by 2030, the spending on Alzheimer's disease will be as much as the total Medicare spending on everything in this country today. This is not a stochastic process. This is not a maybe. This is going to happen, plus or minus a little bit. This situation is best compared to astronomers following a meteor hurtling toward San Diego, aimed to hit a very precisely calculated place and time. What would we do if we had such a situation? I think we would take it a little more seriously than we take the economic meteor that's coming just as predictably our way.

"From a social and economic view," Harry Tracy wrote recently in *NeuroInvestment,* an industry newsletter, "it is about the money, the growing diversion of resources to sustain life in those increasingly unaware of their own lives. There is no greater public health issue looming in the developed world."

When pharmaceutical companies decide what diseases to pursue, they look at the daunting numbers. The market for possible neurodegenerative disease therapies is simply too huge to ignore. So it was with ampakines. No matter what difficulties Cortex faced, the prize was potentially too great to give up.

Ampakines, regardless of their ultimate fate at the hands of the FDA, have been in existence long enough, and seemed promising enough, that they have taken on an existence separate from Lynch and Cortex. Other companies have licensed certain formulations of the drugs for certain disease indications, or have developed their own versions, but, probably more important in the long run, the drugs have found a constituency within the academy.

University scientists are by and large desperate people. They live under almost constant threat of annihilation and thus are always on the hunt for novel approaches to long-standing problems, approaches they can use to make discoveries, get published, win grants, and win tenure. (There are, by one estimate, a mere twenty thousand tenured professors of biology in the entire United States. But the universities confer more than five thousand biology Ph.D.s annually. These people have nowhere to go and no money to get there. The average age of a biologist winning his or her first principal investigator grant has increased to forty-two. In other words, a scientist is likely to be in midcareer before winning a program grant large enough to support even a modest lab.) The competition is so intense that the only way forward for those not at the forefront of their fields is to search for long shots around the edges. Lynch and Cortex regularly field requests from scientists scattered around the globe seeking small quantities of ampakines to use in their own experiments. This is common practice within academic science and Lynch is usually eager to cooperate. So was Cortex, which holds the licenses for most ampakine iterations and has the final say over who gets the drugs. In practice, the more labs work with your drugs, the greater the chance of success. It multiplies the manpower being applied to the drug development.

Significantly, too, other researchers have broadened the field in which the ampakines might play a role. The AMPA receptors on which the ampakines are designed to act are present throughout the central nervous system and are by far the most common receptors in the brain. In practice, this means the potential targets for the drugs are more numerous than a tiny company like Cortex, or the combined Lynch and Gall labs, can investigate. Without the work of other researchers, the targets for ampakines will necessarily remain limited.

One of the most promising areas of research outside scientists have begun investigating is a rare disease known as Rett syndrome. Rett (or RTT) afflicts very young girls almost exclusively, although there have been rare cases of boys with the disease. It is caused by a mutation in a single gene that is crucial to development and maturation. The mutation interrupts development with utterly devastating consequences. Rett victims appear to be normal, healthy babies at birth and through their first year or two of life, at which time the first symptoms appear. Rett was not a disease Lynch had ever even heard of.

According to the International Rett Syndrome Foundation:

The age when RTT begins and the severity of different symptoms may vary. The child with RTT is usually born healthy and shows an early period of apparently normal or near normal development until 6–18 months of life, when there is a slowing down or stagnation of skills. A period of regression then follows when she loses communication skills and purposeful use of her hands and slowing of the normal rate of head growth become apparent. Soon, stereotyped hand movements and gait disturbances are noted. Other problems may include disorganized breathing patterns which occur when she is awake and seizures. There may be a period of isolation or withdrawal when she is irritable and cries inconsolably. Over time, motor problems may increase, while interaction and communication, especially with eye gaze, seizures, and irregular breathing may improve. Most individuals with RTT require maximum assistance with every aspect of daily living. . . .

Apraxia, the inability (or reduced ability) to program the body to perform motor movements, is the most fundamental and severely handicapping aspect of RTT. It can interfere with every body movement, including eye gaze and speech, making it difficult for the girl with RTT to do what she wants to do. Due to this apraxia and her inability to speak, it is very difficult to make an accurate assessment of her intelligence. Most traditional testing methods require her to use her hands and/or speech, which may be impossible for the girl with RTT. Her mobility may be delayed and she may have difficulty crawling or walking.

Rett children often live for decades, but as captives in their own bodies, which they cannot control. They are frequently unable to do even the most basic tasks for themselves. There is no prospective treatment.

A Rett researcher at Case Western University in Cleveland has given a high-impact ampakine to a mouse engineered with the RTT mutation and essentially cured it.

In Alberta, Canada, another enterprising researcher has investigated the use of ampakines to rescue patients who suffer respiratory depression brought on by opiate-based pain-relief medications after they have undergone surgeries. During their episodes of respiratory depression they are unable to breathe. When such depression occurs, as it does among somewhere between 10 percent and 20 percent of patients receiving opiate-derived pain relief, hospital workers (assuming they become aware of the problem) have no recourse but to take away the medication. The crisis is thus averted, but the patient must face recovery in excruciating discomfort. In the worst of cases, the respiratory depression is not noticed until it is too late; the patient dies.

The Canadian researcher determined that ampakine injections resolved the depression and allowed the resumption of the painkillers.

Other researchers are examining a potential role for ampakines in diabetes care. In Lynch Lab, Eni Kramar came back to the lab on weekends to work with Julie Lauterborn from Gall Lab on Fragile X, the most common form of mental retardation. The work went so well, she returned full-time to the lab not long afterward. She had been making much more money at her industry job, she said, but was bored stiff. Along with the Fragile X investigation, she began an inquiry into cognitive decline among menopausal women.

The fact that so many neural deficiencies can be viewed through the prism of LTP and ampakines has led Lynch, slowly, carefully, to ponder how it is that the presumed substrate of memory is implicated in so many nonmemory activities. "I now suspect," he notes, "that many diseases involving memory-cognition defects will ultimately screw up the theta-integrin-BDNF–actin polymerization–shape change–synapse change–LTP process. They come at it from different directions, but at some point mess it up. This probably means that the LTP process is the most complex thing neurons do in a short time frame. The process is the weak link. But I think there is more to the story, just don't know what."

The combined Lynch and Gall labs have been turning out so much work that Lynch often finds himself buried in the data, trying to convert it into words and the words into publishable work. It is a measure of the labs' success that someone as prolix as Lynch is at times unable to keep up. He loves doing the data analysis—it is a form of escape and learning. He'll dive like a solitary swimmer into the pool of numbers and sink down among them, happily losing himself in the murk. His writing process is similar, although the farthest thing from enjoyable—it is torture. Lynch often starts writing a paper very early in the run of a project. It is a way of clarifying an hypothesis and organizing the plan of attack. It tells him what he has and what he lacks and will need. He had the cofilin paper mapped out in his head before Chen and Rex produced the data to support it. This means, among other things, that he is constantly waiting for the real world, as it is experienced out on the lab benches, to catch up to the explanation of the world he is building in his computer.

Over the years he has persuaded himself he can assist his writing by drinking. Typically, he'll write through the day, and when he hits what seems to be a wall in the evening, he breaks it down with booze. He'll sit there at the Mac late into the night, night after night, sipping whiskey. "Just me and Mr. Jameson," he'd say. He also chews on cigars. He can't smoke them without setting off his bronchitis, so he extracts the nicotine by chewing it into mulch.

These periods can be accompanied by communication blackouts—no telephone or e-mail, very little contact with anything outside the numbers. He is attached to his computer, chained to it, it seems, for weeks at a time. Sometimes when I stopped by to see him during these periods, it would take some time for him to emerge from the data dream in which he was immersed. He would look up when I entered the room; he could see me, but it wasn't clear he knew who I was, and he couldn't immediately speak. It was as if he were reemerging on a foreign shore and needed to determine what language was spoken there. He was always hospitable to me, despite the interruptions. He wasn't so kind to others. He resented intrusions that, he said, were costly in terms not just of lost time but of lost ideas. The process of seeking coherence in the data and fitting it into words and the words into prior hypotheses is delicate and prone to collapse without sustained attention. A single telephone call can cost him hours.

For reasons no one, least of all Lynch, can explain, at this moment he agreed to coauthor a book for a general, nonscientific audience, something he had long wanted to do. Except the book wasn't about LTP or cognitive enhancers. It was about a long-forgotten episode in the history of African paleontology and its relevance to brain evolution. The venture produced a quirky, incisive, ambitious, fascinating book (called *Big Brain: The Origin and Future of Human Intelligence*) but also created a whole new class of people for Lynch to alienate. His coauthor was Richard Granger, the computer scientist with whom he had done neural-network-modeling work in the 1980s. They got into a dispute about how ready the manuscript was for publication. Granger and the editors were ready to roll; Lynch thought they weren't far past the first-draft stage. He worried belatedly that investing time and energy, both real and psychological, in the book was hurting the lab, which was, as always, at a crucial point.

"About to start surge number two, but got that great mistake dragging around after me like Marley's chains," he said of the book. By the time of publication, Lynch and Granger were barely speaking. The same applied to Lynch and his editor. Their final communications were handled through lawyers. Lynch ended up paying his attorneys more than he earned in royalties.

Lynch also spent considerable time helping to prepare a defense of his ampakine patents against claims made in Europe by Eli Lilly, the Big Pharma company. Europe has its own patent system, distinct from the American process. The two systems generally agree in their results, but prospective inventors have to go through both systems to protect their inventions. The European system is somewhat more vulnerable to challenge, and Lilly took advantage of that vulnerability to file its claims against the ampakines. Lilly argued that the European patent courts should not have granted Lynch and Gary Rogers a patent for invention of the ampakines. The company did not dispute that Lynch and

Rogers had invented the drugs; its main claim was that ampa-kines were so obvious that it took no act of creativity to think of them. Unanswered by Lilly was how it so happened then that no one else had actually made the invention. In a weird way, it was a validation of ampakines' potential utility. Lilly wouldn't have been fighting over the drugs if it thought they weren't viable. The action was a gamble for Lilly, but one with obviously huge potential payoff. Except for the legal fees, which were consider-able but barely a scratch on the bottom line of a company like Lilly, the patent challenge was a free shot. For Lynch, it was a giant pain in the neck.

The LTP work in the lab, the ampakine battle with the FDA, further ampakine research both at Cortex and in the lab, the book, a patent suit, the normal hassles in dealing with the uni-versity, and the Philadelphia Phillies (suddenly a respectable team in a genuine pennant race) all demanded attention that Lynch had no choice but to give. It was a full plate, but appar-ently not full enough. Lynch launched a job search, making quiet inquiries around the country about moving his lab, which would of necessity require moving Gall's lab too. Finding a university with that kind of money available seemed almost impossible. He did a quick tour of prospective employers, giving talks in each place, as is the academic custom. The talks amount to advertise-ments for the science and the scientist, exactly the sort of thing Lynch had long eschewed. Surprisingly, he loved it now. He dis-liked the travel but loved the attention. The most promising des-tination was a new program being built in South Florida by the Scripps Research Institute. Scripps had a long-established and widely respected neuroscience program in San Diego and had raised money to build a similar center in the East. Florida, with heavy state backing, had won the competition, and ground was being broken on the new institute.

Scripps sought out Lynch, and he flew to Florida for conver-sations. They went well. The organization, except for its location, had everything Lynch wanted—great facilities, money, and ambition chief among them. For a man who hated disrupting his routines so much that he frequently canceled long-planned speaking engagements at the last minute simply so he wouldn't have to leave his lab, the idea of unwinding forty years of associations and habits and packing off to the swamps of South Florida was unattractive; but Lynch was disgusted with the UCI administration and intrigued by Scripps. As the discussions continued into the summer of 2007, I published a series of stories about Lynch and his research in the *Los Angeles Times*. The stories sought to portray him as he was, which necessarily included some not-very-flattering descriptions of his habits, his personality, and the trail of strained personal relationships he left behind him. That proved the end of the job talk forthwith. Someone at Scripps informed him that the stories provided "a vivid, perhaps too vivid, description" of his work and life. Scripps, they wrote, is not a stodgy place, but . . .

BUILDING *N*, FALL 2007

Since the first behavior experiments using Chen's new markers, now more than a year ago, the labs had been running and rerunning the experiments, building *n*. Every experiment was, to Lynch, a risk to the entire enterprise. When he viewed the first results, he had commented, "Obviously unbelievable, but highly significant." He progressed from there to "biggest result in the history of memory research." To: "The *n* is now large enough, you don't jump away from it. It's probably true." Then: "Flat fucking unbelievable." Finally: "It keeps me awake at night. Will I be able to lead the children of Neurozion into the promised land? Will I get there myself? Will they build another golden calf?"

In the fall, as if to reward Lynch's fundamental faith that the universe is organized to screw him, the FDA announced it was denying Cortex's request to renew clinical trials for ampakine treatment of ADHD. The ruling came out of nowhere. The resumption of ADHD trials was assumed to be a matter of mere paperwork. Instead, on October 11 the FDA informed Cortex that since there were existing medications already approved to treat ADHD, the agency would not approve further trials for CX717 for that indication. (This was a long-standing FDA policy for any new chemical entity, or NCE, the agency's term for a new drug. The problematic aspect in this instance was that the existing ADHD medications, almost all of which were stimulants, were not that great. Being stimulants, they had significant side effects and the FDA had recently required several of them to print dire, so-called black box warnings on their packages, stating that suicidal ideation might result from taking them.) Cortex executives and Lynch were stunned. Once again the bottom dropped out of the stock price, which sank to below a dollar a share. Analysts had been predicting that once Cortex escaped the FDA's jail, the stock would rise to as much as ten dollars a share. By the time the stock price quit sliding, the company's market capitalization had fallen by more than $200 million in eighteen months. One analyst characterized the FDA action as "abject surrender to timidity." He wrote that the FDA "operates by this motto: 'The only good NCE is a dead NCE.' "

Lynch was devastated. "Got to admit, it hit me harder than might be expected," he said. His depression didn't last long. Cortex immediately began planning to start trials in Europe for the respiratory depression indication that the Canadian researchers had been working on. Several companies other than Cortex had ampakine variations in development. Lynch reasoned that if the drugs worked, and they were safe, at some point they would prevail. Everything between here and there was mere detail. He just wished Cortex and the FDA would get on with it.

The disconnect sometimes seemed bizarre. Life in the lab was a victory feast. The ampakines were marching through neural diseases like Lynch's beloved Roman legions. Outside, in the world of money and men, Cortex was scrounging emergency rations. Every time the company advanced a mile, it was ambushed from the rear. Lynch did what he usually did when faced with a hostile environment—he ignored it. Partly this was a rational choice. What else could he do? Obsessing about the difficulties of Cortex would not alleviate them. Partly too it is simply the way Lynch approaches scientific problems. He likes to strike the tents and head for the high country. Once there he will worry about whatever scattered wreckage might be left behind.

This pattern had started with the seminal 1984 paper, "The Biochemistry of Memory: A New and Specific Hypothesis," and continues up to the present. The recent behavioral paper, "Evidence That Long-Term Potentiation Occurs Within Individual Hippocampal Synapses During Learning," made the logical but nonetheless staggering claim that LTP is memory. Ever since it went to the printers in July, Lynch had been anxiously awaiting his comeuppance. Speaking of the behavior paper months after it was published, he said:

> Notice that these uncertainties did not stop us from charging ahead with the model building, and writing papers with strongly stated hypotheses. Doing so is scary. This is why confirmation of the basic hypothesis from different angles is so important to me—why the reaction to confirmation is never "Well, sure, that's what we expected." Confirmation from different approaches lets me ignore, for now, those things I can't explain, ignore the clear evidence that the overview is incomplete.

This strategy isn't selfless. Lynch is always highly competitive and fearful of losing credit for discoveries. He makes bold hypotheses in large part to establish his priority. The long-standing case against him—that he stretches the bounds of his science to make overly ambitious claims—is sometimes right in the narrow sense that he makes the most ambitious claims possible, not always supported by the evidence on offer. But the critique is wrong in its fundamental implication, that he ignores the evidence that doesn't fit. If anything, he does the opposite.

He spends years backtracking through every possible route looking for ways to test his claims. That he does this, and that others leave it to him to do, says much about the way contemporary biological science operates. Everyone is a free agent, every result a one-off. Conversations and even formal presentations at the various symposia reflect a peculiar intellectual disaffection. New findings don't build one upon another but are often scatter-shot. Sometimes (usually if they deal with a disease or a gene that is said to cause a disease) new findings with very little credibility rise above the din, then just as quickly fall back into the ambient noise. You can publish anything, right or wrong, pedestrian or provocative, and nobody blinks. Every other week newspapers and magazines run stories based on the latest paper that claims to have identified the memory gene or the politics gene or the Alzheimer's gene. They come and go, rarely remarked upon, almost never remembered. Many of these announcements undoubtedly deserve to sink, but that raises the question of why they were ever published in the first place. And what happens when genuine discoveries are made? Lynch's behavioral paper stated as forthrightly as possible that LTP is memory. There is no other way to read it. He declared the century-long run over, the riddle solved, and demonstrative proof provided. And what happened? Almost nothing. Barely a squeak of recognition or even complaint. The circumstances recall a famous formulation by the geneticist J. B. S. Haldane: "Theories have four stages of acceptance: (1) this is worthless nonsense; (2) this is an interesting, but perverse point of view; (3) this is true, but quite unimportant; (4) I always said so."

Maybe, as UCLA's Alcino Silva has said, the field has lost the ability to even recognize, much less contest, Newtonian-scale achievement in its midst. Lynch is inclined to blame the loss of ambition on fear and careerism, but there seems something deeper at work. The broad, almost giddy early excitement of the 1970s gave way, in turn, to the retrospectively too-arrogant optimism of the 1980s, then the federally designated assault of the 1990s Decade of the Brain. The excitement dimmed as it came up against the hard targets of the brain and was replaced by a kind of niggling incrementalism across the field; people gave up hope that such a thing as big discovery was even possible.

CHAPTER THIRTEEN

"So we come to another one of those jump-off-the-cliff moments"

MAPS, 2008

One day in early 2008, Lynch, his usual embattled self, remarked, "It's an odd thing, but the pressure feels greater than ever before. Can't figure it."

This feeling might have been simple, well-oiled paranoia, earned over decades of intense competition, but it was contrary to the general tenor of his current circumstances. Lynch had swept the board clean over the past several years, and what stakes remained seemed lower. On the basic science of LTP, his competition had largely melted away. Others working in the field were more likely to cooperate than contend. Rex went off on separate trips to Alabama and England to consult directly with collaborators. Kramar was working with Wyeth, the pharmaceutical company, on her menopause investigation. Lynch, when he spoke at scientific seminars, was often besieged by offers of collaboration. He gave a talk to a convention of neurologists and told them, in his description, that "a great simplification regarding diseases of memory and cognition was about to come banging on your doors at three a.m. Of course, they ignored this preposterous statement and wanted to know, instead, when they could get ampakines for their own experiments." He also joined a consortium funded by, of all things, Las Vegas casino money, to investigate the use of ampakines for treatment of brain and spinal injuries.

Even things that were by definition combative evaporated. In

January Lynch flew to Munich for the big European patent throw-down with Lilly's lawyers. Almost as soon as he was seated in the witness chair, Lilly moved to have him blocked from testifying. The judges allowed the motion but in the end granted only the smallest of Lilly's claims and allowed Cortex's patent to stand, pending resolution of appeals. It seemed effectively the end of the effort to revoke the patent. "The thing was a joke," Lynch said. "Ninety minutes later I'm racing to the *Flughafen* [airport]." He was home in Irvine by midnight and back in the lab by morning.

He and Gall pieced together a proposal for a national engram-mapping project that, as envisioned, would involve as many as ten or twelve other labs.

The end of the research on consolidation (the persistence data) had left but one final undertaking—the maps. Mapping the changes that occur during learning would effectively end the LTP chapter in brain research and open up vast new areas of exploration. All prior debates about LTP's artifactual status would be moot, taken aloft, as Lynch would say, in the giant blimp and dumped somewhere in the Pacific trench, forgotten. Maps would bring the science into the real world. More than that, memory maps ought to provide insight into the way the brain actually works, where it puts things, how those things are used. "To be specific," Lynch said, "what do you do with an engram once you actually have one? Ask how the scattered parts are pulled into coherent action—recall and thought."

Alcino Silva agreed: "We still don't know how the brain works. We know memories are distributed in all these structures, but we don't understand how the structures compete, what synergy they have. We don't understand the rules. One of the first steps to understanding them is identifying the areas, visualizing them. Once we know where, then we can ask how are they coordinated, related, etc."

Mapping had gone into limbo—put aside, not abandoned—

when the phalloidin staining method proved too transient to be useful. The biggest hurdles to resuming work on it had been, first, sheer manpower—there simply weren't enough people in the lab to work the problem—and, second, everything else had gone so well in the interim that there was little sense in slowing down those projects. In short, the success of the science had interfered with the mapping. Eventually, though, those successes reinvigorated the mapping too. As seems to happen more often than not in the lab, the success of one project feeds into another. Chen's success in finding more long-lasting and later-stage LTP markers provided new tools for making maps.

Rex took over the engram project, plus everything else he could get his hands on, and decided the lab could never succeed in building a map if all of the steps were done manually. The main steps included: training animals in specific tasks; staining the brains after the training so that the locations of the things the animals had learned—the memories—could be observed; and surveying the brain tissues to find those markers. Of these, there was really no conceivable way to accomplish the training and staining other than the way they were currently being done. That left the final stage—surveying the tissue and recording where changes occurred. This was a mammoth undertaking.

In the original phalloidin experiments, Lynch tried to demonstrate that LTP changes synapses and that these synapses can be marked. The scientists had done this with synapses in the olfactory cortex, an area Lynch was very familiar with from previous work. Looking in one place and finding what you are looking for is an utterly different undertaking from finding those same changes throughout the entire cortex. To have even a chance at success of making maps, researchers would have to survey the huge brain expanses of every trained animal. Recall that even a rat likely has more than a trillion synapses. To have any chance at success, Rex believed, this step had to be automated. He wanted a system in which slices of brain tissue, after they had been stained, could be systematically scanned and photographed with the microscopes and the results immediately fed into computers for analysis. He tried a few commercial software packages that purported to do exactly this, but they were all too slow, too inexact, too inefficient, or all three. He decided to write his own program, but found it much more complex and time-consuming than he had anticipated. Given Lynch's normal demand for a breakneck pace in all things, mapping kept getting pushed down the priority list.

Rex eventually began the tedium of writing the new program, which would automate sampling and measurement over broad swatches of tissue. The main challenge was to develop a system that accurately balanced the light signals from the fluorescent stains. The microscope could sample only at so many elevations in the tissue, while the actual marked synapses would be scattered at different elevations. The practical effect was that some stains were brighter solely because they were at the surface of the brain tissue, while others were buried more deeply. The varying brightness had to be normalized, or it would corrupt the analysis. Rex spent four months on the light balance issue alone.

At the beginning of the coding, he thought he could accomplish what he wanted with one relatively simple software routine. It ended up requiring more than one hundred subroutines. "The thing was becoming a scientific marvel in its own right," Lynch said. "Nothing like this exists elsewhere."

Once Rex got the program up and running, Chen and another grad student joined the project to help. Rex networked six different computers to do the data analysis, and as a sample task, they began mapping the entire rat hippocampus.

They used the same learning task the group had been employing for their LTP and behavior experiments: naïve rats (Kaspar Hausers all) were allowed to explore a new environment for thirty minutes. They used two sets of control animals: one that was never allowed into the learning environment, and a sec-

ond that was allowed to explore but was first injected with a drug
that blocked the NMDA receptor, presumably blocking LTP.

By mid-September, the project was finally at full speed. The
first set of six rats was trained and sacrificed, their brains
extracted, frozen, and labeled with the fluorescent dyes. The
hippocampus of each animal was divided according to a grid of
three hundred sections. Each section was photographed through
a microscope. The photography alone took ninety minutes per
grid. The level of data being accumulated was massive. Producing a finished image of the entire hippocampus required 4,200
individual images, each of which was itself a computer recon-
struction of five separate images. Recall that a rat hippocampus
is about a quarter-inch long and less than one-eighth of an inch
deep.

The results from the first sets of animals were unexpected. As
Lynch is fond of saying, big results always are. The encoding was
highly selective and densely clustered throughout the hippocampus. No one had anticipated the clustering effect, but the
first pair of experimental brains to be analyzed had exactly the
same sort of clusters. They were in different places in the hippocampus, but they were very much alike in the volume and distribution of overall staining. The control animals that had never
been allowed to explore had nothing remotely comparable. And
the control animals that had been in the experimental environment but with their NMDA receptors blocked had maps virtually identical to those of the other nonexploring controls. This
result tied into twenty years of experiments showing that blocking the receptors blocks LTP. Here it blocked memory. It was a
powerful indication that fit the long-standing hypothesis that
LTP is the basis of memory.

Rex, blasé as ever, was intrigued, but nothing more. "It could
be the greatest fluke ever," he said. He was nonetheless sufficiently impressed that he gathered up the data and the images
and went over to IOI Theory to show Lynch.

Lynch was alone in his office, writing, when Rex knocked and said, "I've got something to show you."

The images were loaded into Lynch's computer, called up, and displayed. Lynch took one look and his head snapped back. He had a funny, almost fearful look on his face. "Are those what I think they are?" he asked.

"They are what you think they are," Rex replied.

"Holy shit," Lynch said, then repeated it slowly. "HOOO-LEEE SHIT. It's in clusters."

"So far," said Rex.

Said Lynch, "That's bye-bye to the constraints inherited from a half a billion years of randomness. . . . Great pictures. Great pictures. Those will look great on the cover of *Science*. Give me two more, and that's where it will be—the cover of *Science*."

Lynch was off to the races, immediately drawing up a new experimental paradigm to determine how different the maps might look using previously trained rats. "Do sophisticated rats use a tiny fraction of synapses to encode new information relative to the bozos we're now studying? We'll look at the frontal cortex at last."

The clustering effect wasn't the only differentiation revealed in the experiment. Each neuron appeared to have encoded memory differentially on its own dendrites. All the marked synapses appeared to be in the apical dendrites (those that grew out of the top of the neuron). There was no marking in the basal dendrites (those that grew out of the bottom of the neuron).

The two sorts of groupings—one across the hippocampus and one within each neuron—suggested that memory is not randomly encoded, as had been long assumed, but follows some sort of organizing rules. In this sense, the results fit with the neural-network models that Lynch and Granger proposed in the 1990s. The basal-apical dichotomy echoed differences Chen had found just weeks earlier in LTP experiments. It appeared that LTP occurs very quickly, actually, in the basal dendrites, but is never consolidated; it is wiped clean before ever stabilizing.

Talking about it then, Lynch had said:

The idea of post-learning shaping of memory is novel. If it is tied to oscillations—sharp waves, theta pulses—then the whole idea of learning will have to be broken into two phases—acquisition and shaping—with both under the control of entertaining variables. . . . The basal-dendrite stuff and mossy-fiber results suggest the brain is breaking up the memory problem and assigning the parts to different anatomical systems. In other words, the idea of continuous uniform memory is a perceptual illusion, something produced by brain.

The next day, Lynch was still taken aback by Rex's result. In an e-mail, he wrote:

Long time ago I suggested to you that the first memory maps would change everything. Couldn't say why (a surprise) but here it is. Basal dendrites and clusters.

If we accept it, then we'll be on to another place.

He followed up later:

The NMDA receptor blocker results are conclusive and freak me out. Wouldn't trust it except that:

1) It's exactly what happened in the Vadim [behavior] paper and

2) Lulu has the same effect in her pilot study on BDNF signaling.

Just so hard to accept that it's as simple as this—that encoding of long-term memory is pretty much LTP.

So we come to another one of those jump–off–the–cliff

moments. Been a few of these over the past three years: phal-loidin works and says that TBS [theta burst stimulation] triggers the formation of actin networks; actin networks con-solidate LTP; synapses get bigger with LTP; learning pro-duces the same effects.

And now, with the Rex results, everything converges on neural-network models saying that LTP-based synaptic learning rules will not only encode long-term memory but shape its organization into mathematically definable pat-terns. And then there's the basal dendrites not having any modified synapses. A second memory system for transient info.

Fuck 'em. I'm buying it, and once more into the breach, dear friends.

THEORY 101

Lynch, when he talks about LTP, often illustrates his points by drawing diagrams as he goes along. He will take a fine-tipped pen and make arrows and lines to show the direction of currents, and variously shaped boxes and squiggles for different mole-cules. He labels everything in a tiny, careful script.

In its simplest form, this was helpful for me in gaining some rough understanding of the relationships among all the many moving parts. But as time went on, the sketches grew ever more elaborate, sometimes ending in an action-painting explosion of inked lines darting here, there, and everywhere on the page. It didn't always make things clear, but it was certainly helpful in disabusing me of my high school biology notions of relatively straightforward and simple cellular functions—here's the cell, here's the nucleus, this happens, then that. Indeed, a tally of the proteins, enzymes, and other molecular actors involved in mem-ory offered a powerful counterargument to my old model. Seth Grant, a neuroscientist at the Sanger Institute outside London, has counted more than one thousand proteins present at the average synapse. If only half that number were actually doing something, isolating and understanding the behavior of each of them would be a herculean undertaking. Lynch was prosaic about the complexity. "It's a bitch and two-thirds," he said. "And stupid too."

Even within this convoluted, multivariant world, LTP is a preposterous idea. It is a fabulously complicated process involving hundreds of individual proteins interacting within a space far, far smaller than the head of a pin every time it occurs, which is to say, hundreds of proteins are engaged by the second. To think that the whole point of that whirlwind of activity is to slightly alter the shape of a tiny portion of a tiny cell, to relax its surface and thus allow room for more molecules of a very particular type to emerge from within the cell—and that's how memory occurs? If you were not a biologist, the whole notion might seem a seriously crackpot idea. Ingenious, yes, but crackpot. It is actually more evidence of the degree to which human biology is the result of millions of years of evolution and random mutations, some of which have served useful purposes and some of which haven't. Evolution has had a direction, Lynch liked to say, and it isn't toward perfection. Over time the useful mutations have survived. The process is far from elegant, and the resulting organism is a magnificent contraption, a sackful of accidents stuffed with extra parts and sometimes contradictory actions that nonetheless work. Well, much of the time.

Brain scientists, better than almost anyone, see in their experiments the routine evidence of biological complications. The mammalian brain is very much not how you would have designed the thing if you had started out with a clean slate. If you could, it is highly unlikely you would use the molecules that heal scratches on your arm to secure your memories, but no one was in charge of this process.

You might compare it to building a computer operating system. The two best-known designers of operating systems are Apple and Microsoft. Apple's software is highly praised for its intuitive design and simple elegance. Microsoft, contrarily, is criticized for its bloated, all-things-for-all-people messiness. Its operating systems are routinely decried as kluges, not built from the ground up but patched together out of existing parts, only some of which worked well in their initial iterations. Microsoft doesn't do this because its software engineers are idiots. Its kluginess owes in large part to the corporate decision to make its operating systems as backward-compatible as is practically possible. Apple, valuing its aesthetics over its customers, often goes back to a clean slate. Sadly for us, we are all PCs. Our operating system was very definitely not built from the ground up. Evolution by definition is backward-compatible. The design of our brains has evolved, adding new features every million years or so, but we've been stuck with a lot of the old features too, and probably some mutations that never worked very well but stuck around nonetheless. We are compromised, full of repurposed parts, always building on top of what was already there. The human brain, by any definition, is a kluge. It's amazing it works at all.

Lynch had in his career tried hard, he thought, even if no one shared the opinion, to remain modest, shying from ideas that were too big or theories that reached too far. He had thought it vain to suppose he could formulate an overarching explanation of the brain. Now he wasn't so sure. Was he now standing in a place from which he could reach at least the low branches of the tree and shake it to see what fell to the ground? Lynch began trying to fit the LTP story into a bigger picture. How much brain biology could be folded into it? A physicist, when grandiose, will talk about devising a TOE—a Theory of Everything. Lynch wasn't quite ready for that. This was still biology, after all. Most often, he said he would settle for a TOAL, a Theory of a Lot. On his more optimistic days, he sometimes aimed higher still, to a Theory of a Lot More.

Such a theory would start with the olfactory cortex as a model for the mammalian brain. Small mammals engage the olfactory system, as it happens, by sniffing. And not just random sniffing, but sniffing at a particular rate—about five times per second, the theta rhythm. If, as Lynch believes, the olfactory system became the model for the human neocortex, one of the things that came with it was the sniffing rhythm. "The rhythm's there, so it got co-opted," he said.

For years theta's primary role was seen as opening the AMPA and NMDA receptors, but during the disease investigations, Lulu Chen determined that the BDNF receptors are also affected by theta. Not only does theta initiate LTP, it creates the optimal conditions for its success. "I find that extremely spooky," Lynch says.

> That's the moment I begin to think that maybe this is close to a Theory of a Lot. That tells you there's been a powerful selection pressure toward this rhythm, and it's pulling more and more into it. . . . In the hypothesis of the future I'm going to suggest that this thing goes a lot further—the shape of dendrites, the shape of cells—by needing to use this rhythm for encoding of information, that cells, fifty million years of evolution later, have found out that they're stuck with this rhythm. Even though they're no longer olfactory animals. It's too fucking bad. Even primates that have almost no olfactory cortex, they're still stuck with this, can't back-track. . . . It's a real argument against there being a designer. No designer would do this.
>
> What happens is you go along with this, and some fucking thing pops out—this is what exaptation is, something pops out—that there was no selection pressure for it at all. It

was never selected. It was just there. And all of a sudden some animal went like that [he snaps his fingers] and realized they could use it for this. You backtrack from this and say, "Wow, this was the biggest and bestest thing that ever happened to that goddamn animal." There wasn't any reason. It was just the dumb junk you piled into the system over and over again, and guess what? Some of it happened to be useful.

You just pile all this crap in here because you go, "I wanted this." There's this selective pressure for something else, and it puts this patch on it, and then you did this kluge, and then you did that, and all of a sudden: Boom! Whoa. Wait a minute. Hoooo! That's the story. It's the origin of everything we talk about. That shit fascinates me. I think it's elegant. I think it's complete science, and I think it has tremendous intellectual ramifications. But there again, this perfectly captures what's wrong with me in the neuroscience world. Because they don't give a fuck at all. If I go to a convention and say, "This rhythm, listen—" "Okay, the dumb fucker wasn't satisfied pretending to be a chemist, we accepted that, but this, oh god." They don't want to hear a word of it.

Is there any reason they should? Perhaps there wasn't back in the 1980s, when Lynch first began talking about theta. It was important, yes. The optimal rhythm for initiating LTP in the laboratory? Okay. But who needed all of this exaptation mumbo-jumbo? Lynch wasn't 100 percent certain himself. But some clues were beginning to emerge from the detailed LTP examinations of the past year.

We now have three signaling phases following TBS [theta burst stimulation]. The first goes from a few seconds to several minutes, the second from 1.5 to 10 minutes, and the third from 7 to maybe 60 minutes. It is very, very weird that you can stack things up across time like this in the tiny volume of a spine head. Step one generates potentiation. Step two assembles the actin filaments. Step three stabilizes them.

Lynch had been obsessively focused on getting to that final step, determining what it is that in the end stabilizes LTP and hence memory. He tended to regard any failure to stabilize as just that—a failure. Indeed, when he looked at a variety of cognitive disorders, he saw the LTP process falling apart over and over again, not always in the same way, but falling apart all the same. Another way of phrasing that would be to say that when LTP fails, a disease condition is present.

There had been, however, a whole string of results that didn't fit this model: Chen's quantum spines, most obviously, but also some that were less dramatic. LTP, in some instances, persists but doesn't stabilize. That is, you can reverse it almost at will. Why is that? There is no evident condition that causes it. It just happens. And not all of the cognitive failings, even in the various diseases, are primarily memory disorders. Some involve other aspects of cognition. If LTP were solely a device for making memories, why would its breakdown affect other cognitive activity?

The implication is obvious. LTP is involved in more than memory, and what Lynch had always regarded as the failure of LTP might not be failure at all. Richard Morris, the British neuroscientist who had collaborated with Lynch on and off for years, had critiqued this aspect of Lynch's thinking—that he was obsessed with determining how perceptions are converted and stored, how they are made to last. Morris felt this was too single-minded, ignoring as it did the question of why we take in so much and remember so little. Morris wanted to know what happened to cause all the other stuff to be discarded. "I have the opposite mental reflex to Gary. Gary wants everything to last," he said. "I want everything to go away."

Most everything does go away. Unlike popular metaphors for memory—say, a video camera—we record very little of what our eyes see. What is the stuff that doesn't go into memory? Lynch was now forced to consider these questions more seriously.

"Time is a big problem for the brain," he says.

> Behavior takes several seconds—synapses operate in the millisecond range—and the ends have to be tied to the beginnings. Continuity of thought may depend on LTP processes. Of course, the whole thing can only work if there are ways to (a) encode LTP without stabilizing it—there are—and (b) get rid of it—the reversal effect. . . . We don't have anything approaching a good idea what a thought is. You ask, what is consciousness—we neuroscientists have a clue. Using the discoveries from the basic biology, we are now beginning to map memories. Once we begin to map memories, we'll begin to figure out how they're assembled. Once we figure out how they're assembled, we'll start to get an idea of what thought is.

Encoding memory isn't the point of every cognitive activity. LTP is initiated by a particular rhythm of action potentials. Action potentials are the main thing the brain does. Those that aren't involved in LTP likely aren't just the brain spinning its wheels, although that is possible too. The concepts that we call thought, cognition, consciousness, and memory are obviously related. You can't have memory without the others preceding it. Gerald Edelman, a Nobel laureate biologist who has devoted the second half of his career to the study of consciousness, has elegantly captured the nature of at least a portion of the relationship by describing consciousness as "the remembered present."

Lynch, reluctant at first, has begun to edge out onto the reedy shore of this new mystery. There seems to be just too much activity to signify nothing. Once there on the shore, of course, Lynch dives in. Consider, he says, "the vastly complicated problem of temporal integration." He uses writing as an example.

> When writing, you got the sentence being juggled, the paragraph that's supposed to have some point, the overall idea in the head, and then all the rules for writing. There are specialized devices for some of this, but the great bulk of it has to be done within the active networks. Time in seconds, minutes, and longer. All of this is mediated by changes in synaptic strength, LTP being induced and erased, moment to moment, across colossal numbers of networks. It's the continuity and temporal integration that the LTP machine is handling. Memory is the wrong word for all of this . . . it's thinking.

This train of thought would never have seemed feasible to Lynch had the lab not gone into such detail on the timing and the chemistry of LTP and if that work hadn't led to the disease investigations. "I would never otherwise have seen that possibility," he says. "Odd, isn't it?"

Lynch's project for twenty-five years had been trying to determine whether LTP, a laboratory invention, had any relevance to the real world. The Lynch and Gall labs had developed a view deep into the LTP process that suggests it is central not just to the encoding of memory but to much more. Although no one—including Lynch—had ever dreamed of this possibility, it made intuitive sense. Neurons are not fixed entities. They are live cells operating in a complex, dynamic, ever-changing environment. The brain is virtually always doing something. Signaling, initiated from the environment or internally, is constant. Lynch has come to believe that Chen's discovery of quantum spines (so called by Lynch because they seem to randomly move in and out of potentiated states), while a part of the mystery, is also a clue to its solution. They make the most sense if considered as part of a time continuum.

"Maybe you need that quantum, fully reversible LTP to keep circuits active long enough to move across behaviors," Lynch said, guessing that "quantum LTP adds temporal continuity to actions; it bridges the millisecond range of brain operations to the seconds–minutes range of behavior and thought. LTP that we know and love is part of a much larger story."

Perhaps, he said, "consciousness emerged when continuity of brain operations extended into the many-seconds range," that is, "when memory became so dense, and interconnected, that the brain noticed that it, the observer-generator, was always absent from the incredibly detailed pictures."

Lynch, by framing his LTP inquiry in a particular way and not abandoning it until it was finished, had at times put himself at the margins of his field. He was all too aware that others—even friends—relegated him there, but he had hewed to what he regarded as the fundamentals. He bet big. He was rewarded. He had gone searching for memory and eventually found it. And he found the basis for a theory of thought in the bargain. Not a bad bet.

The writer Raymond Carver used to tell fellow writers that their first obligation is to do their work, to, as he put it, be at their station so that if the big ideas, the great stories, ever come along, they will be available to write them down. It is in some sense a simple matter of dedication and perseverance. Stay at your station, he advised. Lynch had, by any measure, stayed at his station. He had done more. He had chained himself to the mast.

In midsummer 2008 Lynch sent me this e-mail: "Finally showed that chronic ampakines reverse disease-related memory problems."

Followed within a week by this: "We've now got solid evidence with new markers that the increase in synapse size is still present one hour after theta bursts. Been waiting a long, long time for this moment. So that's the end of the end of the road."

Another month after that he told me that Rex's engram project would just about bring all of science to a halt.

It took me years to realize it, but I finally had to admit to myself that Lynch would never reach the end of the road. He would never be done. Going back through four years of conversations, e-mails, and telephone calls, I find that the most typical comment from Lynch is a proclamation that soon—in a few hours, a couple of days, a week, a month or two, within the season, by the end of the year—the science would be done. He would reach a plateau, a realization, an end, and he would then stop. Somehow, however, no matter the plateau upon which he found himself elevated, the end never came. The plateaus were but stepping-stones. The science that flowed out of the labs never stopped flowing.

I had signed up for a few weeks, maybe a month or two. At the end of the first year, I believed him when he said the end was in sight. I began to doubt this by the end of the second. As I write this, it is nearing the end of the fourth year, and Lynch is still in there at IOI Theory, the noise of neuroscience debates a barely discernible low hum in the distance. He's inside, still swinging the hammer, still trying to break the rock, to reveal the code that surely lies within.

The nature of science is that it doesn't stop. Ever. The road has no end. The nature of Lynch is that he won't stop either. It seems fitting, somehow. Despite his many protestations to the contrary, he won't stop until he has beaten the thing to the ground. Knowing that is not possible, he goes on anyway, acting as though it is. Some days—often, actually—he is the only one there at the lab. He sits alone, frequently sick as a dog, the doors locked, no phone, no e-mail, not even a name on the door to betray his presence. The only way you would know he is there at all is the blue 'Vette out front and, of course, the science, which, no matter the circumstance, difficulty, or hour, has poured out of him for thirty years like water from the well. And it pours still.

Afterword

The project I had originally come to Lynch Lab to observe—a discovery program aimed at creating maps of memory, or engrams, as they were sometimes called—had provided the lab entrée to a whole new world of science. Through the engram search, which stuttered, shook, and sometimes stopped entirely, the scientists had finally fallen upon a path down which they glimpsed the astonishing world of the synapse in greater molecular detail than had ever seemed possible. So they slogged on. And, as seldom happens in science—or any human pursuit— their dreams were exceeded. In hundreds of experiments over a period of five years, they found evidence to provide a new and detailed description of that synaptic world and the molecular machines that construct it.

The engram project itself, however, was left behind. Chris Rex, who had taken it over, had too little time and attention to devote to it. Even when he was able to concentrate on the mapping, the technical difficulties remained daunting. The team had underestimated the sheer number of obstacles the project faced, and overcoming them required huge increases in computing power and microscope time. New, more durable equipment had to be located. Software had to be written or rewritten. Technical skills had to be developed.

When Lynch's team initially started the project, they were using a piece of equipment called a confocal microscope which, because it can be focused at varying depths in a slice of tissue, was excellent for building pixel-by-pixel three-dimensional images of synapses. The confocal worked beautifully and produced stunning images down to the scale of a single dendrite, but because the confocal images were built from thousands of separate images, they were dreadfully slow to construct. Studying a single synapse wasn't a problem, but the mapping project contemplated surveys of hundreds of millions of synapses across the entire hippocampus. The confocal was simply too slow and provided too much detail. They switched to an optical microscope, with which Rex had presented his initial pilot study to Lynch in the fall of 2008. His results, both fascinating and counterintuitive, had shown what appeared to be clusters of activated synapses in particular regions of the hippocampus. If the pilot result held up, it would mean the mammalian brain had somehow evolved rules for sorting seemingly random data.

Earlier, Rex had automated as much of the project as he could, writing computer code to direct the scanning of the microscope and then the analysis of the data, which allowed the microscope to work unattended for hours at a time. Unfortunately, the successful implementation of this yielded a new failure. The microscope was not rugged enough for such continuous work; filters kept burning out from the prolonged exposure. Rex switched equipment again and, working with the optical company, Leica, customized a new microscope that protected the filters. Data gathering became fully automated, except the microscope now produced too much material to analyze quickly. So Rex brought in a computer programmer to examine what he had built and see if there was a way to speed up the data analysis. Rex said the programmer, Jeff Shelley, "professionalized" his coding. Shelley said it was not so much professionalization but parallelization that was needed.

"There was a bottleneck and it was definitely a CPU not a memory bottleneck," Shelley said. "It was just a way of throwing more workers at it." He rewrote the code so that the data could be directed to as many computer processors as Rex could string together. Effectively, this meant the data could be analyzed as quickly as the rats could be trained. By the end of 2010, the process had been optimized to the point that data which had taken several weeks to analyze could now be read in seven or eight hours.

Once the machine started cranking out data, it became clear that the pilot study had been dead-on. The clustering effects held up. Which is not to say they made any sense. Whole swaths of the hippocampus showed almost no activated synapses, but in certain areas, the enhanced synapses were in clusters; then the deeper you looked, in clusters of clusters. Seemingly random inputs yielded structured results, something for which "there is no known biological basis," Lynch said. Self-organizing systems are not unknown in biology but explanations for them are hard to come by. "Nobody on this planet knows of any anatomy that would produce this clustering. Everything we know about this would have predicted random distributions. We're not seeing that. Where does this pattern come from? That's problem number one."

In trying to address this, the scientists were once again plagued by the limited duration of the markers they were using to see the synaptic changes. To view the changes, they tagged certain molecules with fluorescent dyes knowing that those molecules appeared at the synapse only if the synapse had been activated during LTP. The molecules they had been using for markers—cofilin and a kinase named PAK—had themselves been chosen because they were present somewhat longer than other molecules at the synapse after it had been activated. Still, they disappeared within thirty minutes. Lynch wanted something more durable. One obvious candidate was the type of molecule upon which Lynch's whole theory of memory construction was based—integrins. Recall that integrins are used throughout mammalian biology to tie structures into place after changes have been made. The most obvious example was the role integrins played in healing wounds. Integrins stitch together wounds to stop bleeding, and it turned out they did something similar in the brain. Once the microstructures of neurons were sliced apart then rebuilt during memory formation, integrins tied the newly rebuilt structures together. If they were doing this, Lynch asked, they had to last, right?

He assigned Alex Babayan, Rex's heir apparent as alpha male graduate student, to see if the integrins themselves could be used as markers. What Babayan discovered was perplexing. A particular type of integrin was surprisingly transient. It appeared at the synapse then disappeared relatively soon— within ten or fifteen minutes. Babayan determined that the integrins were turned off for a period, but returned in force an hour after their first appearance.

Lynch had long assumed that LTP, once initiated by theta burst stimulation, was as strong as it would ever be. It had an on/off switch and couldn't be naturally enhanced after its initial occurrence. John Larson, who discovered theta rhythm's role in LTP in the 1980s, had tested what might happen if more bursts were delivered after the first stimulation. He tested at various intervals up to thirty minutes and found it made no difference. LTP was an all-or-nothing affair. But looking at Babayan's integrin experiments, Lynch recalled that psychologists persistently reported that learning occurred best when students were allowed time between learning trials. It had been established that learning was most effective when students were exposed to new information not randomly, but at approximate sixty-minute intervals. This is commonly referred to as spaced learning in the psychological literature. It is far more effective than continuously repetitive instruction delivered every five to ten minutes. Again, no one knew why.

When Larson found no difference up to half an hour after the first stimulation, Lynch had told him to stop testing. If it wasn't going to be enhanced in the first thirty minutes, it was probable it would never be enhanced, he had thought. Now Lynch wondered if he had stopped Larson too soon. He asked Eni Kramar to do a quick, basic LTP experiment to see what would happen if a second set of theta burst stimulation was applied sixty minutes after the first. To his astonishment, she reported a huge increase from the LTP baseline. It nearly doubled.

"If I had done that experiment twenty-five years ago, the whole field would have had an entirely different history," Lynch said. "All these years, I've been working with 50 percent of the effect—arrrrghh . . . This raises the possibility that optimal learning requires spacing of presentations by about the length of a classroom session. We are checking this, but the results point to a biological explanation for one of the key elements of learning theory—spaced trials work better than massed ones. "

A member of a review panel looking at the data later stated the finding "will clearly revolutionize our understanding of core learning and memory phenomena." Another reviewer said the experiments yielded "evidence that the entire field of synaptic plasticity has been striving for since the first description of LTP in the mid-70s."

Lynch began a collaboration with a virtual reality lab in San Diego that was putting human subjects through an analogue to what the rats faced in the unsupervised learning mazes Lynch's team had constructed in Irvine. The human subjects were outfitted with sensors that measured neural excitations in different areas of the brain as they faced simulated, new, complex environments. Lynch hoped to match the human results in spaced learning trials with the memory maps obtained from the rats.

In some sense, this brought Lynch back to where he had begun. When he had entered the field of neurobiology in the early 1970s, he was fleeing what he felt was the eternal squishiness of psychology. He wanted hard scientific results and thought biology could deliver them. There had at the time been no genuinely useful hypothesis for how memory was formed. As Karl Lashley had written, "in spite of such evidence against it," it was clear learning occurred, memories were made. No one had a clue why. By now, most, although still not all, scientists in the field agreed LTP was a—if not *the*—mechanism for making memories. The accumulation of experimental LTP evidence— much of it from Lynch's lab, still more from other researchers around the globe—seemed to fit precisely with what was known about the psychology of learning. The spaced learning experiment was yet one more result. It was becoming more difficult by the day for the resistors to hold out. Almost forty years after it had been discovered, LTP had arrived.

Acknowledgments

Thanks foremost to the members of the Lynch and Gall labs at the University of California, Irvine, especially to Gary Lynch, Christine Gall, Eni Kramar, Chris Rex, Lulu Chen, Danielle Simmons, Laura Colgin, Julie Lauterborn, Ted Yanagihara, and Vadim Fedulov. This book would not exist without their generosity of time and spirit.

The original reporting for much of the material here was done for a series of articles that appeared in the *Los Angeles Times*. That reporting would not have occurred without the support of Dean Baquet. The subsequent articles would not have been published without the assistance of Roxane Arnold and the editorial intervention of Doug Frantz. Thanks to them and others at the *Times* who helped with the series, in particular to Leslie Carlson, whose illustrations were a treat for readers. Thanks to the American Association for the Advancement of Science and to the Wistar Institute for honoring the *Times* articles as part of their annual awards.

Thanks to Larry Swanson for careful reading of early versions of the manuscript and expert guidance through the thickets of neuroscience.

Thanks to Edward Kastenmeier and Tim O'Connell at Pantheon.

Thanks to Paul Bresnick.

Thanks as always to my family, who tolerate (barely and with unfounded hope that the results will be somehow worthwhile to us all) my interests and the absences they entail.

Glossary

ACTIN: A protein that forms a critical part of the interior scaffolds that give cells their external shape. Think of the internal tubing that supports a tent. From the outside, you see only the tent's fabric, but its shape is determined by the interior scaffold. Actin changes form slightly, and once it has formed the scaffold, it is said to be polymerized.

ADENOSINE: A molecule that exists throughout mammalian biology. In the brain, it appears to perform a specific function in the memory process—erasure.

AMPAKINE: A class of drugs designed to enhance communication between brain cells. If they work as envisioned, the drugs, still in development, would enhance almost all cognitive activities.

CEREBRAL CORTEX: The "gray matter," the topmost part of the human brain, wherein complex functions such as memory, learning, and thinking are accomplished.

DENDRITE: A fiber that extends in bunches from a neuron. Dendrites receive signals from another sort of fiber called an axon. Dendrites and axon meet at the synapse.

DENTATE GYRUS: A portion of the hippocampus. Lynch Lab found that a natural electrical rhythm, known as sharp waves, originates here. Sharp waves, the lab hypothesized, are a means by which the brain erases things it does not want to commit to long-term memory.

GENES: Strings of DNA that form a blueprint from which the

organism is built. Each gene contains instructions for building a particular protein.

HIPPOCAMPUS: A cortical structure near the center of the brain in mammals, including humans, that is involved in memory, learning, timing, and spatial awareness, among other functions.

INTEGRIN: One of the most common types of molecules in mammalian biology, integrins mainly function to tie things into place. For example, they cause blood cells to clot, thus allowing wounds to heal. Lynch Lab hypothesized that integrins solidify LTP, locking the molecular changes into place.

LTP (LONG-TERM POTENTIATION): The strengthening of connections between brain cells that occurs when they communicate, making subsequent communication more likely. The communication consists of electrochemical exchanges between two neurons at the synapse, which is where they meet.

NEURON: The most common type of cell in the brain (numbering approximately 100 billion). LTP occurs between two neurons.

NEUROTRANSMITTER: Molecules that are released from an axon across the synapse to a dendrite's receptor. Specific neurotransmitters pair with specific receptors.

NEUROTROPHINS: A family of molecules that promote the growth and survival of neurons.

PHALLOIDIN: A toxin derived from mushrooms. Its use in the biological sciences owes to the fact that it binds to polymerized actin protein. Phalloidin can be stained with fluorescent dyes, and when infused into cell populations, it sticks to the actin, thus becoming a marker for the actin's presence. Scientists can then look at the cells and, by locating the fluorescent stain, determine where actin polymerization has occurred.

PHYSIOLOGY: The study of biological function.

PROTEIN: Molecules that perform most of the work within a cell. Each protein's composition, and thus function, is dictated by a gene.

PSYCHOLOGY: The study of the human mind and behavior.

RECEPTOR: A molecule on the surface of a cell that acts as a sort of docking station for other molecules, including neurotransmitters.

SHARP WAVE: A naturally occurring brain rhythm that originates in the hippocampus and seems to erase LTP. In other words, it causes forgetting.

SPINE: The nubby point on a dendrite where it contacts an axon. Each dendrite has thousands of spines.

SYNAPSE: The point where two neurons communicate. It is actually not a structure but a gap of about 20 nanometers (20 billionths of a meter), across which one neuron sends chemical signals that are received by another. The chemicals set off cascades of events inside the receiving neuron. The human brain contains an estimated 100 trillion to 10 quadrillion synapses, allowing for immense memory capacity.

THETA RHYTHM: A mid-frequency, naturally occurring rhythm in the brain—about four to six cycles per second—that is hypothesized to initiate LTP and thus memory.

Selected Bibliography

Kandel, Eric R. *In Search of Memory: The Emergence of a New Science of Mind.* New York: Norton, 2006.

Kandel is one of the great figures of twentieth-century neuroscience. This autobiography covers a great deal of the significant science of his time.

Lane, Nick. *Power, Sex, Suicide: Mitochondria and the Meaning of Life.* New York: Oxford University Press, 2005.

Intriguing ideas about cellular life and death and the aging process.

LeDoux, Joseph. *Synaptic Self: How Our Brains Become Who We Are.* New York: Penguin, 2002.

LeDoux is an accomplished neuroscientist; this book is among the most accessible of those written from within the neuroscience community.

Levitin, Daniel. *This Is Your Brain on Music.* New York: Dutton, 2006.

This extraordinarily informative and accessible book, written by a neuroscientist who was formerly a record producer, examines the neuroscience of hearing, but it is applicable to the larger issues of brain functioning.

Linden, David J. *The Accidental Mind: How Brain Evolution Has Given Us Love, Memory, Dreams, and God.* Cambridge, Mass.: Belknap Press of Harvard University Press, 2007.

Perhaps the single best contemporary book on the brain for general audiences. Informative, whimsical, and smart.

Lynch, Gary, and Richard Granger. *Big Brain: The Origins and Future of Human Intelligence.* New York: Palgrave Macmillan, 2008.

Writing the book nearly killed Lynch, but it's an entertaining, instructive, and intelligent investigation.

Schacter, Daniel L. *The Seven Sins of Memory: How the Mind Forgets and Remembers.* Boston: Houghton Mifflin, 2002; and *Searching for Memory: The Brain, the Mind, and the Past.* New York: Basic Books, 1997.

Schacter, a memory researcher, is the premier popularizer of the psychology of memory, of which these books are good examples. Psychology is essentially the science of the mind as viewed by its behavioral results; neuroscience is an attempt to understand the brain from its underlying biology.

Shenk, David. *The Forgetting: Alzheimer's: Portrait of an Epidemic.* New York: Doubleday, 2001.

An excellent survey of the scope of the dementia problem and research aimed at combating it.

Swanson, Larry W. *Brain Architecture: Understanding the Basic Plan.* New York: Oxford University Press, 2003.

An insightful primer on how the brain is constructed and what its architecture implies.

Tanzi, Rudolph, and Ann Parson. *Decoding Darkness: The Search for the Genetic Causes of Alzheimer's Disease.* New York: Perseus, 2000.

A first-person account of the search for the presumed genetic roots of Alzheimer's disease.

Thompson, Richard F., and Stephen A. Madigan. *Memory: The Key to Consciousness.* Washington, D.C.: Joseph Henry Press, 2005.
These two eminent neuroscientists provide a straightforward history.

The National Library of Medicine has an excellent Web site on memory: http://www.nlm.nih.gov/medlineplus/memory.html. So does the Alzheimer's Association: http://www.alz.org/index.asp.